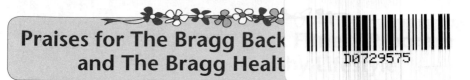

Praises for The Bragg Back
and The Bragg Healt

These are just a few of the thousands of testimonials we receive yearly, praising The Bragg Health Books for the rejuvenation benefits they reap – physically, mentally, emotionally and spiritually. We look forward to hearing from you also.

Thanks to Paul Bragg and Bragg Health Books, my years of asthma were cured in only one month with The Bragg Healthy Lifestyle Living!
– Paul Wenner, Gardenburger Creator • *www.gardenburger.com*

When I was a young gymnastics coach at Stanford University, Paul Bragg's words and example inspired me to live a healthy lifestyle. I was twenty three then; now I am over sixty, and my health serves as a living testimonial to Bragg's health wisdom, carried on by his dedicated health crusading daughter, Patricia. Thank you!
– Dan Millman, Author "The Way of the Peaceful Warrior"
www.danmillman.com

Paul Bragg saved my life when I attended Bragg Health Crusade in Oakland. I was so weak and sickly, that I had to wear a back brace to sit up. I thank Bragg Healthy Lifestyle for my long, healthy, active life and I love spreading health and fitness.
– Jack LaLanne, Bragg follower since 15 • *www.jacklalanne.com*

As a youth I had a learning disability and was told I would never read, write or communicate normally. At 14 I dropped out of school and at 17 ended up in Hawaii surfing. My road to recovery led me to Paul Bragg who changed my life by giving me one simple affirmation to repeat: "I am a genius and I apply my wisdom." Paul Bragg inspired me to go back to school and get my education and from there miracles happened. I have authored 54 training programs and 14 books and love to crusade around the world thanks to Paul Bragg.
– Dr. John Demartini, Dynamic Crusader
Star in "The Secret" • *www.drdemartini.com*

For 35 years I've followed The Bragg Healthy Lifestyle - It teaches you how to take control of your health and build a healthy future.
– Mark Victor Hansen, Co-Creator, "Chicken Soup for the Soul" Series

Good health and good sense are two of life's greatest blessings. – Syrus, 42BC

Our prayers should be for a sound mind in a healthy body. – Juvenal

a

Praises for The Bragg Healthy Lifestyle

Thanks to the ageless Bragg Health Books, they were our introduction to healthy living. We are very grateful to you and your father.
– Marilyn Diamond, Co-Author "Fit For Life"

Thank you Paul and Patricia Bragg for my simple, easy to follow Bragg Health Program. You make my day!
– Clint Eastwood, Bragg follower for over 50 years

Bragg Books were my conversion to the healthy way.
– James F. Balch, M.D., Co-Author, *Prescription for Nutritional Healing*

The Bragg Healthy Lifestyle, the Bragg vinegar drink and fasting has changed my life! I lost weight and my energy levels went through the roof. I look forward to my fasting days. I think better and am a better husband and father. Thank you Paul and Patricia. It's a great blessing in my life. Also, Patricia, we enjoyed your health sharing at our "AOL" Conference.
– Byron H. Elton, VP Entertainment, Time Warner AOL

I met Paul Bragg on April 6, 1964 at the famous "L" Street Beach in Boston. We became instant friends. The following day he introduced me to his daughter Patricia. We have been friends ever since. Both Paul and Patricia have always been health inspirations to millions around the world, but especially to me! I gave my first public lecture with Paul and Patricia in April of '64, I was 22 then, I am now 63. Paul was always dynamic, energetic and a life-changer! Patricia has continued the Health Crusade and has more energy than any 3 people I know put together.
– Dr. David Carmos, Co-Author with Dr. Shawn Miller
"You're Never Too Old To Become Young" • *perfecthealthnow.com*

Thank you Patricia for our first meeting in London in 1968. You gave me your Fasting Book, it got me exercising, brisk walking and eating more wisely. You were a blessing God-sent. – Rev. Billy Graham

---

Paul Bragg inspired me many years ago with the Bragg book *The Miracle of Fasting* and with his philosophy on health. His daughter Patricia Bragg is a good friend of mine and is also an inspiration and testament to the ageless value of living the Bragg Healthy Lifestyle. I love the Bragg product line and am still inspired by the many books Paul and Patricia have written.
– Jay Robb, Clinical Nutritionist, author *The Fruit Flush 3-Day Detox*

b

Praises for The Bragg Healthy Lifestyle

I have been consuming Bragg's Apple Cider Vinegar consistently now for only 4 months, 3-4 times per day. My lower back aches and hip pain are totally gone from 25 years of jogging and martial arts. Like your book says, "try it and you be the judge." Well I've tried it and I will always purchase it. I love it. Thank you.
– Kelly Numrich, Saskatchewan, Canada

The Bragg Healthy Lifestyle, vinegar drink and brisk walking (3x daily) for 20 minutes after every meal, helped eliminate my diabetes! My whole body, circulation, feet and eyes have all improved. Thank you, may God continue to bless your Crusade. – John Risk, Santee, CA

Bragg Super Power Breathing helps make the weak strong and athletes champions. – Bob Anderson, famous stretching coach *www.stretching.com*

I have been following the Bragg Healthy Lifestyle for about two months. I am on a college student budget so sometimes I have a hard time affording some of my veggies, but I believe in Bragg Books and the Bragg Lifestyle. So far with the Bragg Organic Apple Cider Vinegar I am feeling so much better than I used to . . . all the stiffness in my shoulders and neck is disappearing and I feel so much stronger and energetic. Thanks. – David Meyer, Boise, ID

I read your book on the uses for Apple Cider Vinegar and I am now taking it daily. After passing on the book to my mom, she too started using Bragg ACV and found that the pain in her shoulder that had been waking her up at nights for years has been greatly reduced. It's such a simple thing, but so effective. I am now interested in all aspects of maintaining health naturally. Thank you so much.
– Catherine Cox, Toronto, ON Canada

Bragg ACV is great. The Bragg Vinegar Drink has now become our Life Supporting System and we passionately support it and cannot live without it! We thank you for all the many ways we can use your vinegar with the miracle mother enzymes.
– Yasuko and Hiro Hashimoto, CEO of NEC, Japan

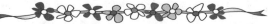

Those with lower back injuries can worsen their pain by avoiding using hurt muscles and its best to trim down if overweight as it increases pressure on spine.
– Newsletter Article from Dr. Mercola. See web: *mercola.com*

c

Praises for The Bragg Healthy Lifestyle

How I beat cancer, obesity, diabetes, strep and three herniated disks and excruciating pain? The answer was changing to the Bragg's Healthy Lifestyle and doing the Super Power Breathing Exercises. It changed and saved my life! I had full recovery and also lost 70 lbs. I received a new life and that is just the beginning because my manhood returned that was lost to diabetes – now that's exciting! On my trip to Honolulu, Hawaii I visited the famous free Bragg Exercise Class at Waikiki Beach. I became so regenerated with a wonderful new viewpoint towards living my healthy lifestyle that I now live in Hawaii. My 6' 2" body is invigorated with new energy for life and living! My new purpose for living is to help others reclaim their health rights! I also want the world to join The Bragg Health Crusade and enjoy super health. I am deeply thankful Paul and Patricia for my new healthy life!
– Len Schneider, Honolulu, Hawaii

I've experienced a beautiful, remarkable, spiritual and physical awakening since reading Bragg Books. I'll never be the same again.
– Sandy Tuttle, Painesville, Ohio

I lost 102 lbs. with the Bragg Vinegar Drink and Bragg Healthy Lifestyle. I have kept it off for over 15 years, exercising and staying away from white flour, sugar and all refined foods. Thank you.
– Dee McCaffrey, Chemist & Diet Counselor, Tempe, AZ

We get letters daily at our Santa Barbara headquarters. We would love to receive a testimonial letter from you on any blessings, healings and changes you experienced after following The Bragg Healthy Lifestyle and this book. It's all within your grasp to be in top health. By following this book, you can reap more Super Health and a happy, longer vital life! It's never too late to begin! Studies show amazing results that were obtained with people in their 80's and 90's – Pages 10 & 28. Receive miracles with healthy nutrition, fasting and exercise! Start now!

Daily our prayers & love go out to you, your heart, mind & soul.
with love,

3 John 2   *Patricia Bragg*   Genesis 6:3

d

Miracles can happen every day through guidance and prayer! – Patricia Bragg

BRAGG
BACK
FITNESS
PROGRAM
with SPINE MOTION
For Pain-Free Back

PAUL C. BRAGG, N.D., Ph.D.
LIFE EXTENSION SPECIALIST

and

PATRICIA BRAGG, N.D., Ph.D.
HEALTH CRUSADER & LIFESTYLE EDUCATOR

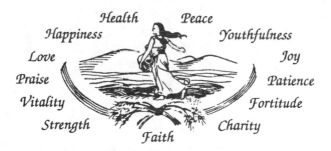

Health   Peace
Happiness   Youthfulness
Love   Joy
Praise   Patience
Vitality   Fortitude
Strength   Charity
Faith

BECOME

A Bragg Health Crusader – for a 100% Healthy World for All!

HEALTH SCIENCE
Box 7, Santa Barbara, California 93102 USA

World Wide Web: www.bragg.com

BRAGG

BACK FITNESS PROGRAM

with SPINE MOTION
For Pain-Free Back

PAUL C. BRAGG, N.D., Ph.D.
LIFE EXTENSION SPECIALIST
and

PATRICIA BRAGG, N.D., Ph.D.
HEALTH CRUSADER & LIFESTYLE EDUCATOR

Health Science, Box 7, Santa Barbara, California 93102
Telephone (805) 968-1020, FAX (805) 968-1001
e-mail address: books@bragg.com

Quantity Purchases: Companies, Professional Groups, Churches, Clubs, Fundraisers etc. Please contact our Special Sales Department.

**To see Bragg Books and Products on-line,
visit our website: www.bragg.com**

 This book is printed on recycled, acid-free paper, which saves thousands of trees.

Sixteenth Printing MMIX
ISBN: 978-0-87790-057-3

Published in the United States
HEALTH SCIENCE, Box 7, Santa Barbara, California 93102 USA

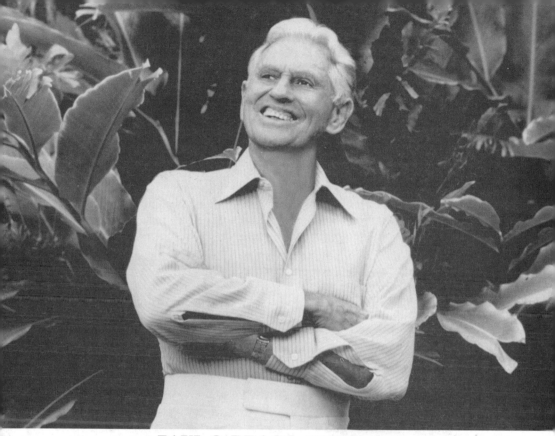

PAUL C. BRAGG, N.D., Ph.D.
World's Leading Healthy Lifestyle Pioneer

Paul C. Bragg's daughter Patricia and their wonderful, healthy members of the Bragg *Longer Life, Health and Happiness Club* exercise daily on the beautiful Fort DeRussy lawn, at world famous Waikiki Beach in Honolulu, Hawaii. Membership is free and open to everyone who wishes to attend any morning – Monday through Saturday, from 9 to 10:30 am – for Bragg Super Power Breathing and Health and Fitness Exercises. On Saturday there are often health lectures on how to live a long, healthy life! The group averages 75 to 125 per day, depending on the season. From December to March it can go up to 150. Its dedicated leaders have been carrying on the class for over 35 years. Thousands have visited the club from around the world and carried the Bragg Health and Fitness Crusade to friends and relatives back home. When you visit Honolulu, Hawaii, Patricia invites you and your friends to join her and the club for wholesome, healthy fellowship. She also recommends you visit the outer Hawaiian Islands (Kauai, Hawaii, Maui, Molokai) for a fulfilling, healthy vacation.

To maintain good health, normal weight and increase the good life of radiant health, joy and happiness, the body must be exercised properly (stretching, walking, jogging, running, biking, swimming, deep breathing, good posture, etc.) and nourished wisely with healthy foods. – Paul C. Bragg

(See Bragg Photo Gallery on pages 123-128)

i

Decades of Amazement As Life Rolls By

Where did our years go? They went by so fast.
When we're young they seem to cra-a-wl,
With each decade, they fly past!

At 29 we're the center; At 30 we feel supreme
But 40 strikes terror; Life's not what it seems.
By 50 we've reached maturity; At 60 we accept seniority.
When we're filled with excitement of creative living,
There's no room for depression and despair!

But at 65, wisdom that comes from experience
Then takes over and we learn to accept ourselves as we are.
Each new day is a gift to be treasured,
Enabling us to go far!

At 75, life is for the living
But it is through our sharing, loving and giving
that we reach the Stars of Joy, Peace
and the Possibilities of Eternity!

– by Ruth Lubin, 88 years young & going strong,
who started writing poetry & sculpturing at 80!
PS: Ruth is a fan of the Bragg Healthy Lifestyle for over 58 years!

PROMISE YOURSELF

- *Promise yourself to be so strong that nothing can disturb your peace of mind.*

- *To talk health, happiness and prosperity to every person you meet.*

- *To make your friends feel that they are special and appreciated.*

- *To look at the sunny side of everything and make your optimism come true.*

- *To think only of the best, to work only for the best and expect only the best.*

- *To be just as enthusiastic about the success of others as you are about your own.*

- *To forget the mistakes of the past and press on to the greater achievements of the future.*

- *To wear a cheerful countenance at all times and give every living creature you meet a smile.*

- *To give so much time to the improvement of yourself that you have no time to criticize others.*

- *To be too large for worry, too noble for anger, too strong for fear and too happy to permit the presence of trouble.*

– Christian D. Larson

WE NEED YOUR SUPPORT!

With Your Support The Bragg Health Institute Can Continue on the Teachings of Paul C. Bragg

For over 80 years we have been sharing Paul C. Bragg's teachings on healthy living worldwide! Millions have followed the Bragg Healthy Lifestyle principles and their lives have been changed forever! Everyday people send us letters, e-mails and call, saying – *"Paul Bragg saved my life!"*

Former U.S. Surgeon General, Dr. C. Everett Koop said Paul Bragg did more for the Health of America than anyone he knew of.

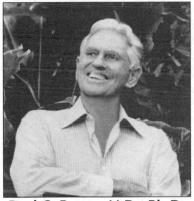

Paul C. Bragg, N.D., Ph.D.
Originator of Health Stores
Life Extension Specialist
Health Crusader to the World

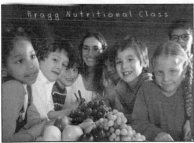

Bragg Outreach to Schools

If your life has been touched and helped by Bragg health teachings, please help us carry on the Bragg Legacy into this 21st Century and beyond. Your tax deductible donation to the *Bragg Health Institute* will support the teachings to continue the Bragg Message of Health to the world for future generations.

The non-profit and philanthropic work of the *Bragg Health Institute* funds The *Bragg Health Crusades*, community health, health education lectures, seminars, and publications on healthy living. The Institute conducts health outreach to youth in schools, organic gardening teaching programs, and helps sponsor health science research and provides scholarships to worthy students pursuing the natural health science professions.

Please join us in sharing The Bragg Health Legacy!

(Please see next page for more information)

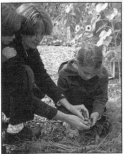

Organic Gardening
Teaching Programs

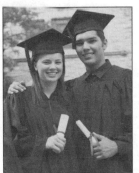

Bragg Scholarships

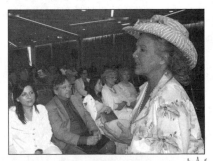

Patricia Bragg lecturing at
Bragg Health Seminars

iii

HEALTH DREAM WITH NEW HEALTH VISION

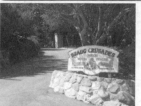 The Bragg Health Institute is located on a beautiful 120 acre Campus and Organic Farm on the coast of Santa Barbara, California. Patricia Bragg and the Directors of Bragg Health Institute have designated this as the future site of the greatest living tribute to the life of Paul C. Bragg. The new Bragg Health Institute will become a world center for organic and healthy lifestyle education and research. (See the *Mission, Purpose and Vision for the Future* Video on *www.bragghealthinstitute.org*)

You can also be part of Paul Bragg's lasting legacy by having your name permanently inscribed upon one of the educational nature walks or inspirational walls that will enhance the natural beauty of the Bragg Health Institute Campus and Organic Farm. Or you may want to have your name inscribed in the Grand Entrance or one of the rooms in the Bragg Memorial Library or Health Education Center. Your 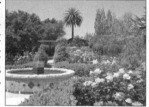 name can be part of your own legacy, as you will be recognized for generations to come as a great Health Crusader because of your financial support of this wonderful health project. When thousands of visitors see your name each year, they will know that you helped make a difference in the world.

Some of the Special Projects for the New Bragg Health Center:

- Paul C. Bragg Memorial Library
- Organic Medicinal Herb Gardens
- Paul Bragg Memorial Rose Gardens
- Bragg Healthy Lifestyle Videos & DVDs
- Cuisine Teaching Demo Kitchen
- Health Eco Education Center
- Organic Teaching Gardens
- Bragg Nature & Farm Walks
- Bragg Health Museum
- Special Events & Programs

— — — — — — — — — — — — *COPY AND MAIL* — — — — — — — — — — — —

YES! I would like to help support Bragg Health Crusades by making a contribution to the Bragg Health Institute, a 501(c)(3) non-profit foundation, tax ID# 27-0983248. Your contributions are tax deductible.

❑ Enclosed is my tax-deductible gift of $_____ ❍ VISA ❍ MC ❍ Discover
  ❍ $25 ❍ $50 ❍ $100 ❍ $250 ❍ $500 ❍ $1,000

❑ Please send me info on where my name can be permanently inscribed at the Bragg Center.

My gift is in memory of or in honor of _____

Please send a note indicating a gift has been made in their memory or honor to:

Credit Card Number:_____

Signature:_____

Card Expires: _____ / _____
month / year

Name _____ **PLEASE PRINT**

Address _____ Apt. No.

City _____ State _____ Zip _____

Phone ( ) _____ e-mail _____

*If giving by check, please make check payable to: **Bragg Health Institute***
Mail To: Box 7, Santa Barbara, CA 93102 USA • (805) 968-1020

For more info check out our web: www.bragghealthinstitute.org

Spreading health worldwide since 1912

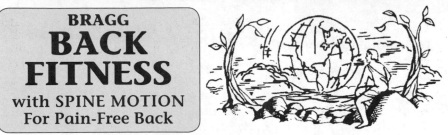

BRAGG
BACK
FITNESS
with SPINE MOTION
For Pain-Free Back

To preserve health is a moral and religious duty, for health is the basis for all social virtues. We can no longer be as useful when not well. – Dr. Samuel Johnson, Father of Dictionaries

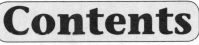

Contents

Bragg Healthy Lifestyle Plan

- *Read, plan, plot, and follow through for supreme health and longevity.*
- *Underline, highlight or dog-ear pages as you read important passages.*
- *Organizing your lifestyle helps you identify what's important in your life.*
- *Be faithful to your health goals everyday for a healthy, strong, happy life.*
- *Write us about your successes following The Bragg Healthy Lifestyle.*
- *Where space allows we have included "words of wisdom" from great minds to motivate and inspire you. Please share some of your favorites with us.*

The Bragg Books are written to inspire and guide you to radiant health and longevity. Remember, the book you don't read won't help. Please often reread our Books and live The Bragg Healthy Lifestyle for a long, happy life!

Contents

When you sell a man a book you don't just sell him paper, ink and glue, you sell him a whole new life! There's heaven and earth in a real book. The real purpose of books is to trap the mind into its own thinking. – Christopher Morley

People who maintain an ideal, trim body weight can lower their risk of heart disease as much as 55%. – American Heart Association

Contents

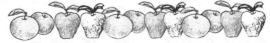

Eating plenty of organic produce – fruits and vegetables – slows down ageing. The ageing under the skin, and chronic age-associated diseases, including heart disease, cancer and degenerative brain diseases, can be slowed down, and even reversed in some cases with a change in diet. Adding lots of fruits, salads, vegetables, onions and garlic, taking vitamin, and mineral supplements and avoiding saturated fats can increase energy and add years to your life. Exercise is also important in delaying ageing. – Nanci Hellmich, USA Today

Contents

Three Needed Health Habits

There are three habits which, with but one condition added, will give you everything in the world worth having, beyond which the imagination of man cannot conjure forth a single additional improvement! These habits are:
* ***The Work Habit*** • ***The Health Habit*** • ***The Study Habit***
If you have these habits, and also have the love of someone who has these same habits, you are both in paradise now and here. – Elbert Hubbard

Contents

Exercising in the Sky – You Arrive Healthier

We even jog while thousands of feet high in the air, soaring skies in an airplane. We go to rear of plane, jog and stretch. We never arrive stiff and tired. Our 70 trillion cells get a massage. Learn to take advantage of spare moments for stationary jog during the day, whether office worker, CEO or housewife. We all need daily exercise for healthy bones, strong heart and a healthy body. Millions are traveling by air, but for people with back pain, air travel can be painful and difficult. Narrow seat widths, more seats being added to pack airplanes to capacity gives less leg and seat space that can cause problems for those who suffer back pain!

Helpful Exercise Tips to Make Air Travel More Comfortable:

• Contact airlines special service department and arrange seating on aisle for more leg room, or bulkhead seat for more comfort.

• Exercises keep your muscles working and prevent back spasms.

• Turn your head to the right, then hold for five seconds and bring back to the front, then repeat to left. Do 5 sets.

• Keep arms by sides and do this shoulder roll - shrug shoulders upward to ears, now roll shoulders back, down and around. Do 5 sets each way.

• Do with shoes off. Lift heels so balls of feet are still on floor, then drop heels back to floor. Now lift up toes, keeping heels on floor. Do 10 sets.

• Walk along aisles and in corridor. Do back arches, by placing hands in small of back and gently arch backwards. Also, do side bends by placing hands on hips and bend gently to right, hold five seconds, and back to upright, then bend to left. Do 10 sets. (See Web: *www.backcare.org.uk/*)

A Perfectly-Aligned, Flexible Spine Is Important for an Active, Healthy Life!

A perfectly-aligned, fully flexible spine is one of the best *head-starts* on perfect health almost all can enjoy! Although we might think that we are born into this world with a perfect spine, it isn't always true! Unfortunately, even as early as the moment of birth itself, the process of damage to the spine has begun. Authorities say that many physicians grab the baby's head as it emerges during birth, twisting the head up and down to bring out the baby's shoulders, stressing and twisting the tiny spine. During this process a number of spinal misalignments and/or slight breaks can happen, interfering with the child's health. This could possibly contribute to sudden infant crib death. Also, if the baby is hung by its feet and slapped on the bottom, a whiplash injury at the base of the skull may occur, causing even more serious damage. Read up on the gentler, more natural childbirth methods that are available in your area.

Further misalignments (known as subluxations) happen during childhood years through spankings, falls, fistfights, and the typical wrenching and twisting of limbs encountered by a normal active child. Sports injuries during the teenage years take their toll on the young spine. As adults, poor eating, sleeping and poor posture habits reinforce all that has gone before, culminating not only in a painful back, but also preventing enjoyment of perfect health. The vital nerves leading from the spinal cord to all other organs in the body haven't ever had a chance to function at their healthy best, because vertebrae have been pressing on them and interfering with their important function. Many times, a general tendency to disease or weak spots in an overall healthy constitution can be traced to such spinal misalignments.

With the simple, gentle Bragg Spine Motion Exercises, many of the effects of a lifetime of neglecting the spine can be reversed dramatically within a few months, weeks, or even a few days! Also, your family Chiropractor can help diagnose and correct most serious spinal mis-alignments that, without your suspecting it, may be adversely affecting your overall health and hindering your natural defenses against disease!

Practicing the easy Bragg Back Fitness Program is the best preventive maintenance efforts for your back health. These exercises and The Bragg Healthy Lifestyle will help you enjoy a flexible, painfree back for life. Remember . . .

You are as Youthful as Your Spine!

Chapter 1

BRAGG
Back Fitness Program
with Spine Motion
For Pain Free Back

Oh! My aching back! This cry has echoed down the corridors of time for countless centuries, ever since humans learned to walk on their own two feet. This unique accomplishment – achieved only by human beings among all the varied forms of mammals on Earth – has given us the mobility and dexterity to cope with any environment found on Earth. It has enabled us to rule all other creatures, to *conquer the Earth* and now to set out and explore outer space.

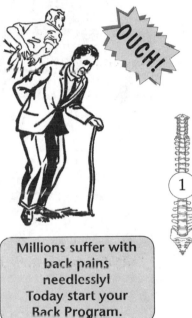

As with almost everything in nature and life, however, there is a price to pay for these accomplishments. Humans are still learning how to stand erect! From babyhood on, every human being repeats the slow learning process – crawler, toddler, walker, runner – and all through

Millions suffer with back pains needlessly! Today start your Back Program.

life must pay attention to their posture and maintain it, or suffer with painful backache and its many related ills.

The Spine Is Your Vital Key to Health

Universal native folklore equates backbone with courage, an intuitive tribute to erect posture and the key role of the spine in physical fitness. However, physical fitness is more than muscular power: It is the superior condition of the human body and its frame.

Practice The Bragg Healthy Lifestyle and these back and spine exercises and practice good posture. An ounce of prevention is worth a ton of cure!

When your body is fit and every muscle or organ is functioning properly, that body becomes a powerhouse of vim and vigor. Physical fitness means more than just plain health and the absence of illness: It means no hidden liabilities and no silent, painless illness working away like termites at the organic framework of your human house. Remember, the spine is the ridgepole of your body – which is your earthly home and temple.

Role of Spine in Human Body

Let us briefly summarize the key role of the spine in almost every function of the human body. It is the pivot of the skeleton – the framework of bones giving the body its shape. Anchored to the spine are layers of large and small muscles and ligaments of the back and abdomen, essential in holding the body erect and the vital organs in place (even these organs themselves are supported by the spine). In four-legged (*quadrupedal*) creatures, vital organs are suspended downward from a curved spinal column. However, in the two-legged (*bipedal*) human, they must be held up against the pull of gravity by an erect, strong spinal column.

In the center of that column, descending directly from the base of the brain and protected by the bony vertebrae, is the miracle spinal cord, the *control center* of extensive, intricate networks of motor and sensory nerves that radiate to all parts of the body (see page 33).

For these basic anatomical and physiological reasons, (which we will discuss in detail during the course of this book,) we believe that many ills can be traced to an abnormal spine. For example, prolonged habits of incorrect posture – as well as accidents, sudden movement, jolt or strain – can cause a vertebra to shift slightly out of alignment (subluxation) and to press against a nerve passing out from the spinal cord through an opening at that level. Such an impingement is an open invitation to trouble in the organ or body part that is serviced by that partially pinched nerve (see pages 29-31).

Of all knowledge, that most worth having is knowledge about health. The first requisite of a good life is to be a healthy person. – Herbert Spencer

For similar reasons, the spine itself is often thrown out of alignment and into abnormal curves toward the sides, front or back of the body. This can adversely affect other bones of the skeleton, shorten or stretch muscles and ligaments, cause organs to prolapse (fall) and/or bring on interrelated malfunctions throughout the body.

Body Misuse Causes Injury Over Time

According to Dr. Thomas G. Gutheil, M.D., Associate Professor of Psychiatry, Harvard Medical School, *There are many reasons for an aching back, a number of which have to do with lifestyle changes, fitness, and the modern environment. Not only does the back carry the body, but it also carries many of the psychological tensions that humans get weighted down with. In my psychiatric training, I learned to look at the posture and body position for clues to a person's mental state: the stooped back whose owner seemed bowed by the weight of depression, the shoulders drawn in and tight, and the head retracted like a turtle's in anticipation of a blow that comes only in the fearful patient's imagination, and the many other posture giveaway signs.*

Sheila Reid, rehabilitation services coordinator at the Spine Institute of New England, observes, *The single event that people think caused their back injury is often not the problem. Instead, it's almost a cumulative trauma. We go through years of back and health misuse, and then there is the one fall or the box or child you pick up that breaks the proverbial camel's back.*

See web: http://www.fahc.org

The ratio of nerves sending messages about our backs, in comparison to the nerves on our fingertips, is much less than a hundred to one! Therefore, we are receiving fewer warning pain signals from our backs. Sad facts: most people tend to ignore their back until it starts crying out to them, calling for help to be relieved of pain and discomfort!

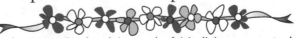

According to the New England Journal of Medicine, one study found that although some back patients were satisfied with treatments provided by back specialists, others are finding good results with alternative therapies like chiropractic care, that cost less, require fewer expensive tests and often solve the back problem with a few simple spinal adjustments. See pages 32, 38, and 117 to 120 for more helpful alternative therapies.

Researchers estimate that a whopping four out of five Americans will experience back pain at some point in their lives. In fact, back pain is second only to the common cold as a reason for visiting a doctor. Annually, nearly 31 million Americans experience back pain, at a skyrocketing cost of $20 billion for medical treatments and disability payments, some on permanent disability!

Our modern machines are taking the place of manual labor, and have significantly deteriorated the physical body over the last 60 years. However, Spine Motion can help alleviate almost any back pain you may encounter and help keep it from decreasing your quality of life.

Bragg Originates Spine Motion Exercises

In order to help alleviate back problems arising from structural spine problems, my father Paul C. Bragg originated the Spine Motion Exercises given in this book.

These exercises were introduced over 70 years ago. Public and press reception were so enthusiastic that claims made by those who used these exercises sounded extravagant. Only a small part of the amazing results reported would have to be true to establish the principle of Spine Motion as the valuable force that it is.

As remarkable as may be the results attained by you and others following these Spine Motion Exercises, we do not want anyone to regard this as evidence that these exercises can supplant all other health measures. They cannot, nor are they intended to do so. You must follow a well-rounded healthy lifestyle program, including proper nutrition, adequate rest and other forms of exercise, all of which we will discuss in this book.

Spine Motion Exercises are also not to be considered a cure for any condition, illness or disease. In fact, nature has no cures, in the generally accepted sense of the word. The human body is self-healing and self-repairing when we work with Mother Nature, not against her. If one feels sick and miserable, it's usually brought on by oneself by failing to obey her God-given natural laws.

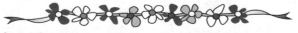

Remember: It's never too late to strive to be what you want to be!
So start to Plan, Plot and Follow through! – Patricia Bragg, N.D., Ph.D.

Paul C. Bragg Recalls
Remarkable Results with Spine Motion

Bragg Spine Motion Exercises are a natural, drug-free approach to health. They are designed to help restore the spine to its natural, normal functions. This helps eliminate the causes of many apparent ailments in the back and other parts of the body that arise primarily from defects in spinal structure. These defects are brought on by poor posture, flabby muscles, improper living and bad working habits or accidents and injuries.

If you are under medical care, do consult your doctor on these exercises and general healthy lifestyle presented in this book. Many orthopedists, neurologists, osteopaths, health professionals (pages 117-120), physiotherapists and chiropractors find this program helpful to their patients.

I have seen back injuries and displacements (having resulted from slips, falls, coughs, sneezes or other sudden movements) respond wonderfully to these Spine Motion Exercises. Occupational accidents, such as sprains, strains or from improper lifting, pulling, carrying or bending, often produce the type of pain and misery that only Spine Motion Exercises can help relieve (plus pages 70 & 91).

At one time, when I returned home from a Bragg Crusade, I found a relative in pain. He had been preparing a piece of ground to plant an organic vegetable garden, and had come across a large, heavy stone. Not realizing how heavy it was, he strained his back while trying to lift it. Unable to continue his work because of severe, crippling back pain, he had been taking all kinds of treatments; however, the condition persisted. I advised him to take hot baths (*add 1 cup vinegar*) daily and, right after bath begin very lightly doing my Spine Motion Exercises. He followed my advice, doing the simpler exercises first, gradually progressing to the more strenuous ones. At the end of one week his pains were gone, and in another week he was once more working in his organic garden.

5

Nature, time and patience are the three greatest physicians. – Irish Proverb

---

Wisdom is the principle thing; therefore get wisdom:
and with all thy getting get understanding. – Proverbs 4:7

I have known cases of severe injuries to the back, such as whiplash from auto accidents, in which great relief was attained by lightly performing simple Spine Motion Exercises. I have also helped many an athlete return to normal after a severe back injury, especially in physically punishing sports like wrestling or ice hockey.

A lifelong athlete myself, I have engaged in all types of sports and my daily practice of Spine Motion Exercises has strengthened my spine so much that I have never had any serious back injuries, despite some bad spills.

Patricia and I receive letters, e-mail, etc. from people all over the world who have followed our instructions in this book and found pain relief from such conditions as lumbago, sacroiliac pain and postural defects of long duration. The exercises have also relieved painful cases of bursitis (inflammation of the bursa, especially of the shoulder, elbow and knee joints), sciatica, arthritis and persistent headaches.

Millions Suffer from a Defective Spine

Researchers have indicated that one in five sufferers of back pain are born with one leg longer than the other. This imbalance can put excessive pressure on the back and spine, the hips and knees. (Try balancing with heel lift.)

About 1 out of 150 persons (of average development) has a sufficiently flexible spine. In today's society, the majority of people are sedentary, warping their spines by faulty posture habits in sitting, standing and walking, by general lack of exercise and improper diet. This applies not only to adults, but also to most schoolchildren who are products of the *TV and computer generation* and of the many schools that don't require basic *physical education*.

A recent study of teenagers in 7th and 8th grade, reports 11% with scoliosis, or spinal curvature. The research was conducted among 841 students in Downey, California, by Dr. Leon Brooks, an orthopedic surgeon in the spine deformity service of Rancho Los Amigos Hospital. Dr. Brooks noted that untreated scoliosis can be responsible for future back pains and respiratory problems. Special exercises are the basic treatment, except in severe cases requiring temporary back braces or, in extreme cases only, surgery.

Spine Motion is Simple and Scientific

Sporadic or incorrect exercise can take its toll on the spine, as overly strenuous exercise, as found among construction workers and some athletes. From the thousands of spine and back cases in our files, **here are three illustrative examples:**

The first case is a person whose spine was so badly slumped that it disturbed his nerve reflexes; he could not take part even in the ordinary play and games of youth. After only four weeks of Bragg Spine Motion Exercises, he became more normally active. Later, he developed into a remarkable swimmer.

The **second case** is of a logger in Northern California who, at age 55, was forced to abandon his rigorous outdoor work due to subluxation of the spine (partial dislocation of some vertebrae). He was puttering at odd jobs around the camp when he started the Spine Motion Exercises. In less than a month, he was able to resume logging. Here was a man who for years had swung an ax, surely a vigorous form of exercise! Even so, the spine had become defective from lack of extension in the right directions and to the right degree. It required the peculiar, anatomical twist of the more scientific Spine Motion to align and flex his spine at every point.

The **third case** is of a 43-year-old woman who was clearly headed for invalidism, with organs supposedly far out of place and ailments that had defied ordinary forms of correction. After a few days of practicing Spine Motion Exercises, she obtained complete relief.

The three cases just described are widely diverse, yet all three responded beneficially to the same Spine Motion Exercises. Why? Remember that the spinal column is the focus of the neuromuscular and musculoskeletal systems. Even a slight dislocation or malfunction in the spine can affect other body parts and cause problems.

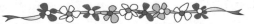

The nervous system falters and suffers when we don't take care of our body.

When recovering from accidents, fractures, etc. it's wise to take extra herbs, and mineral and vitamin supplements to help your body heal faster.

Life is largely a matter of chemistry. – William J. Mayo, M.D.

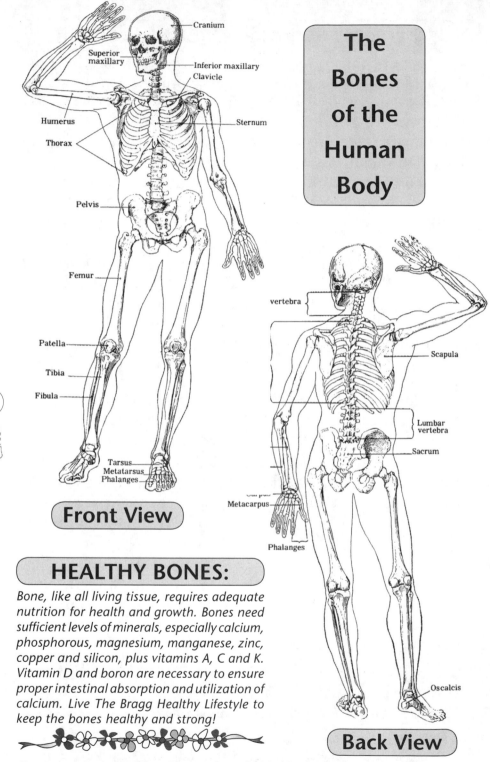

The Bones of the Human Body

Front View

Cranium
Superior maxillary
Inferior maxillary
Clavicle
Humerus
Thorax
Sternum
Pelvis
Femur
Patella
Tibia
Fibula
Tarsus
Metatarsus
Phalanges

Back View

vertebra
Scapula
Lumbar vertebra
Sacrum
Carpus
Metacarpus
Phalanges
Oscalcis

HEALTHY BONES:

Bone, like all living tissue, requires adequate nutrition for health and growth. Bones need sufficient levels of minerals, especially calcium, phosphorous, magnesium, manganese, zinc, copper and silicon, plus vitamins A, C and K. Vitamin D and boron are necessary to ensure proper intestinal absorption and utilization of calcium. Live The Bragg Healthy Lifestyle to keep the bones healthy and strong!

Every man is the builder of a temple, called his body. We are all sculptors and painters, and our material is our own flesh, blood and bones. – Henry David Thoreau

The Spine Works as a Miracle Machine

A scientific study of the spinal structure has made it possible to devise simple spine motions that give your miracle spine the requisite pull or stretch to restore its natural alignment and flexibility. The effects of such motions have been carefully recorded and compared. It has been found that these simple manipulations, through careful, active use of trunk muscles, cause all the tiny bones comprising the spinal column to separate normally and allow Nature to build up the cushiony growths of cartilage between each pair of bones.

Life holds many examples of what resilience means. Imagine an automobile without shocks, a trampoline without springs or a piano without felt hammers.

In thinking of anything mechanical, just recall that every machine ever designed is patterned after the master mechanism constituting the human body. The more perfect the machine, the closer its designers have come to the principles of motion found in the human body.

9

Backs Are Strong if Given Care – Dr. Morris Fishbein

"Fortunately for mankind, the back has developed so well that it is capable of withstanding stresses and strains better than many other parts of the body. There are some who insist that the back is the weakest part of man. Actually, it is one of the strongest. If it could be given the same amount of personal consideration and attention that we give regularly to the teeth, the skin and other portions of the body that are more easily visible, the human back and body would be a more efficient mechanism and would last much longer without breaking down."

– Stated by Dr. Morris Fishbein, Editor 1924 to 1951,
Journal of the AMA (American Medical Association)

Let us explain your spine (the body's mainspring) – its structure and function and how you can give it the loving care and attention it needs to fulfill its built-in potential of performing at least 120 years of good service for you.

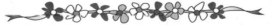

Man's days shall be 120 years. – Genesis 6:3

Conrad Hilton Thanks Bragg for His Long Life!

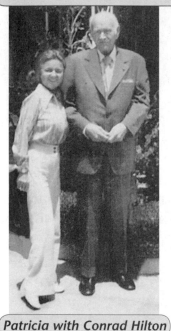

Patricia with Conrad Hilton

When the world's biggest hotel magnate Conrad Hilton was 80 years old and lying on his hospital deathbed, we gave him a new lease on life by introducing him to The Bragg Healthy Lifestyle. He loyally followed our instructions and discovered a whole fresh new healthy, vibrant lifestyle! He was soon healthy, happy and fit, enjoying life! He remained active in business (half days at his office) to almost 100 active youthful years! Mr. Hilton at 88 was quoted in a *People Magazine* interview as saying, *I wouldn't be alive today if it wasn't for the Braggs and their Bragg Healthy Lifestyle!* With this article was a photo of the grateful hotel founder with his healthy lifestyle teacher.

10

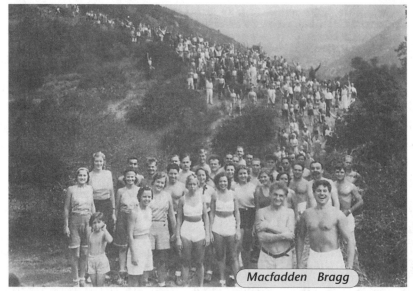

Macfadden   Bragg

A thousand Happy Bragg Health Students Enjoying Hiking, Exercise and Fresh Air on The Trail to Mt. Hollywood, California. Summer, 1932. In the left foreground is Bernarr Macfadden, Father and Founder of the Physical Culture Movement and Publisher of popular Physical Culture magazine and to the right, Paul C. Bragg, Health Crusader and Life Extension Specialist. These Health Pioneers enjoyed leading Health and Fitness Crusades across America.

Chapter 2

Your Miracle Body Mechanic

The Spine and Skeletal System

If you suddenly removed the poles from a circus tent, the tent would collapse. The typical adult skeleton is comprised of 206 bones that support the softer parts of the body and give the body its general shape. If the spine, corresponding to the main pole of the tent, and the other supporting bones (or *poles*) were suddenly removed, the body would sink to the ground in a shapeless mass.

The spinal column, the master bones of the human body, is composed of 26 hollow cylinders of bone called *vertebrae*. If you string 26 spools of thread on a stiff wire in the shape of a very open letter *S*, you've constructed something resembling a spinal column.

The skull, which is supported by the spinal column, is made up of 29 flat bones. The round part of the skull that encases the brain is called the cranium, which consists of eight bones. The face, including the lower jaw, consists of 14 bones. There are three tiny bones in each ear. There is a single bone, the hyoid, in the throat.

The chest is composed of 25 bones: a single breastbone, called the sternum, and 24 ribs. All ribs are attached to the spinal column. The upper seven pairs of ribs (14 bones) are attached to the spinal column at the back and the sternum in front. The next three pairs (six bones) attach only to the spinal column, curve around the front of the thorax (chest) but do not meet the sternum. The two lowest pairs of ribs (four bones), called the *floating ribs*, extend from the spine only partway toward the front. There are two collar bones (clavicles), which are attached to the sternum in front and to the two shoulder blades (scapulas) at each side.

Researchers have discovered the more healthy habits an individual practices, the longer they live and the healthier and fitter they are! – E. Vierck, *Health Smart*

You are what you eat, drink, breathe, think, say and do! – Patricia Bragg

Your Body's Strong, Hard-Working Bones

Each arm consists of one upper arm bone, the humerus, and two forearm bones, the ulna and the radius. There are eight bones in each wrist, the carpi, each with a different anatomical name and function. Five bones, called metacarpi, connect the wrist with the fingers, which are composed of 14 bones, called the phalanges (two in the thumb, three in each finger).

Connected to the lowest part of the spinal column (the sacrum and coccyx) are the two hip bones (coxa), the broadest bones of the skeleton. Each connects with a thigh bone (femur), the thigh bones being the longest, strongest and heaviest bones of the body. In each leg, the kneecap (patella) covers the joint attaching the thigh bone to the two lower leg bones, the shinbone (tibia) and its smaller companion, the fibula.

There are seven bones, the tarsi, in each ankle (larger than those in the wrist). Five bones, called metatarsi, form the arch of the foot, connecting the ankle and toes. As in the fingers, there are 14 bones (also called phalanges) in the toes of each foot, two in the big toe and three in each of the other toes.

12

Keep Your Bones Healthy & Youthful With Exercise & Good Nutrition

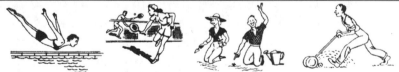

Always remember you have these vitally important reasons for followoing The Bragg Healthy Lifestyle:

- The ironclad laws of Mother Nature and God.
- Your common sense, which tells you that you are doing right.
- Your aim to make your health better and your life longer.
- Your resolve to prevent illness so that you may enjoy life.
- You will retain your faculties and be hale, hearty, active and useful far beyond the ordinary length of years.
- You will also possess superior mental and physical powers!
- By making healthy living an art, you will be youthful at any age.

The Body's Miracle-Working Joints

Except for the U-shaped hyoid bone of the throat, every bone in the body miraculously is connected, or articulates, with another. The spinal column is the main miracle pivot of the entire body skeletal system.

The point at which two bones meet, or articulate, is known as a joint. The joints of the cranium, the part of the skull that houses the brain, are immovable. Those that join the ribs and spine are partially movable. Movement is even more limited in the sacroiliac joints, connecting the base of the spine with the hip bones, where the whole weight of the trunk is supported. Sacroiliac pain (#1 back problem) occurs when the tough, resistant ligaments that hold these joints together weaken under continued or unusual stress, such as lifting a heavy object, a sudden body twist, or the strain from trying to raise a jammed window, etc. (Spine Motion Exercises help strengthen these important ligaments.)

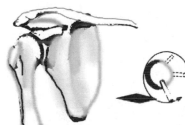

Ball-and-socket joints at hips and shoulders permit freest movement of all body joints.

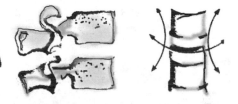

The vertebrae are the saddle joints, moving forward, backward and sideways. One vertebrae moves only slightly on the next, but the whole spinal column is fairly flexible.

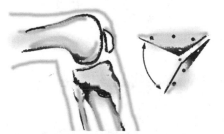

Hinge joints are like the hinges you know – permitting backward and forward movement only – like the hinges of a door. Your knees and fingers are the most used important hinge joints.

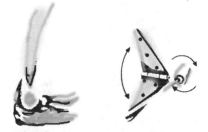

Pivot joints permit the bones to rotate like a key turning in a lock. The elbow is a combination of pivot joint and hinge joint. Thanks to this miracle joint, one bone of the forearm can rotate about the other.

Success depends on your backbone, not your wishbone.

Movable Body Joints – Your Strong Servants

There are four main types of movable joints in the body and, as you will recognize from their names, these human joints have served as patterns that humans have adapted mechanically. Ball-and-socket joints, connecting the shoulder to the arm and the hip to the leg, permit the widest range of movement. Hinge joints, like those of the knees, fingers and toes, allow bending back and forth only. A pivot joint permits the bones to rotate at the joint like a key turning in a lock, such as at wrists and ankles and the joints at the base of fingers and toes.

14

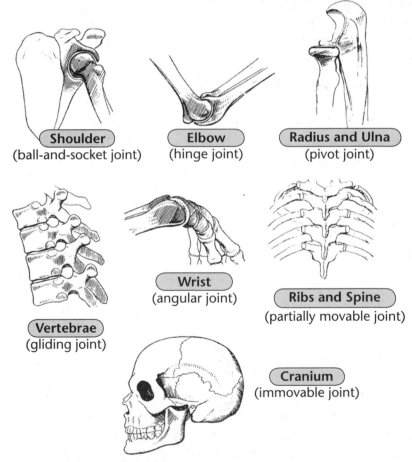

Shoulder
(ball-and-socket joint)

Elbow
(hinge joint)

Radius and Ulna
(pivot joint)

Wrist
(angular joint)

Ribs and Spine
(partially movable joint)

Vertebrae
(gliding joint)

Cranium
(immovable joint)

These are the types of faithful, hard working joints in your body. Between the movable ones, a clear amber lubricant called synovial fluid keeps the joint moving easily. When inorganic minerals from toxic acid crystals or hard drinking water begin to replace this fluid, the joints become stiff, arthritic and painful, and the body feels miserable.

The elbow is a combination of pivot joint and hinge joint, allowing one bone of the forearm to rotate about the other as well as providing a bending motion. *Saddle joints*, like those of the vertebrae, allow movement in all directions that is of a more limited sort than that of ball-and-socket joints. These saddle joints permit limited movement forward, backward and sideways. Although each vertebra moves only slightly on the one adjoining it, the combined movement of the 26 bones make the column rather flexible as a whole.

Nature lubricates your joints with precious synovial fluid, which is permanently encased in a membrane. The natural supply of this fluid is ample for a lifetime, but proper diet is important to maintain its consistency, particularly the avoidance of hard drinking water and other substances containing inorganic minerals, which will be discussed in a later section.

Cartilage – Your Joints' Shock Absorbers

Also lining the bone surfaces of the joints is a tough, springy tissue called cartilage, which not only prevents the bone surfaces from rubbing against each other, but also acts as an all-important shock absorber. This is particularly important in the spine, where cartilage plates and intervertebral disks (described later) between the vertebrae absorb the shocks of ordinary actions such as walking, sitting and blows to the spine.

Cartilage is the precursor of bones in the formation of the skeleton in the embryo, and some of it remains as part of the skeletal system. At birth, the *soft* parts of a baby's skull are cartilaginous to allow room for growth of the brain, changing into hard bone like the rest of the skull after the brain has attained full size. Since cartilage is more elastic than rigid bone, some of it remains at the juncture of the ribs and the sternum to allow full lung flexible expansion. Cartilage also remains part of the adult skeleton in semirigid tubes that must be kept permanently open, such as the larynx, trachea (windpipe), bronchi, nose and ears.

We must always change, renew, rejuvenate; otherwise, we harden. – Goethe

Cartilage, also called gristle, is often confused with tendons and ligaments. All three are tough white tissues with varying degrees of elasticity and differences in structure and functions. *Cartilage is embryonic bone* without a direct blood supply and is semirigid, still somewhat elastic. *Tendons* are the white, glistening fibrous bands that attach muscles to bones. They have great tensile strength but are not elastic. They contain a few blood vessels and sensory nerves. *Ligaments* are of similar structure but contain elastic fibers that connect two or more bones or cartilages and support certain organs, muscles and fascia (fibrous enveloping tissue).

Tendons and ligaments are part of the muscular system, while cartilage is part of the skeletal system. The three are only classified together when dealing with what scientists are now calling the *musculoskeletal* system.

Joints Deteriorate without Proper Care

Many things can go wrong when your joints – and especially the cartilage that cushions them – aren't kept healthy. Besides being more susceptible to injury, neglected joints are prone to chronic conditions such as the many different kinds of arthritis (which means inflammation of the joints). 81.75 million Americans suffer with stiffness, pain, swelling, instability, deformation, dislocation and reduced mobility in their joints. In the United States, over 46 million people have joint problems that can be traced back to damaged cartilage. This damage can result from injury, age, heredity and/or unhealthy living. If you are experiencing severe symptoms, it is important that you consult a health professional to determine the cause and accurately diagnose the discomfort before applying a healing program. In the meantime, there is much that you can do to protect your joints and keep them healthy so that they don't develop problems. And if you do have problems, there are many ways to address them naturally.

Nerve roots are often the cause of low back pain, the second most common cause of missed work days. The back and its problems are the leading cause of disability between ages 19 and 60. Also, it's the number one leading impairment in occupational injuries. Eight out of ten people will have a problem with back pain at some time during their lives. – Medical Multimedia Group

People who suffer from joint problems are often the unhappiest and unhealthiest people. Often they've been taking prescription drugs with dangerous side effects that increase rather than heal their discomfort. Here are some tips for improving their situation.

4 Basic Lifestyle Changes

- *a healthy, well-balanced diet*
- *regular, careful use of herbal remedies and food supplements*
- *use of massage and physiotherapy*
- *exercise and deliberate movement*

1. Balanced Diet: The simple principle is that the more excess weight your body has to carry around, the more pressure there is on your joints and the harder they have to work, producing more wear and tear and eventually, pain! It is commonly known that there is a frequent correlation between being overweight and suffering from varied forms of arthritis. A natural, healthy, toxicless diet not only helps you to keep your weight under control, it also maximizes your body's ability to heal itself. Throughout this book we have more details on how to maintain this healthy life-giving diet.

2. Herbs & Supplements – Nature's Healers: You can actually help heal joints naturally, not just control pain. Because basic symptom of joint trouble is pain caused by inflammation, conventional treatments include anti-inflammatory drugs as aspirin, nonsteroidal anti-inflammatory drugs (NSAIDs) like ibuprofin and steroid drugs as Prednisone. Sometimes a Cortisone injection (caution!) is prescribed for severe inflammation (Braggzyme fights inflammation, page 102). While maybe treatments can be helpful in controlling joint pain, besides being only a quick and often temporary fix, aspirin and NSAIDs are hard on the stomach, intestines, kidney, liver, and actually inhibit the growth of new cartilage!

Your cartilage is miraculously resilient. It changes form when under stress, then springs back to its original shape and with care can be rebuilt and regenerated. Cartilage contains up to 85% water, but the remaining substance includes a wide variety of important sulfur-containing compounds.

Sulfur is essential in repair of cartilage and joints and is in many foods (beans, cabbage, garlic, etc.) as well as supplements. Sulfur is important and necessary for collagen synthesis and to keep synovial fluid rich and nourishing.

Herbs and Supplements have proven helpful in preventing joint disease, reducing pain and restoring injured or inflamed joints. These are available in health and vitamin stores:

• *DHEA Supplement: stands for dehydroepiandro-sterone, a natural substance produced by our adrenal glands. DHEA decreases with age and is linked to age-related joint discomfort, as well as the loss of mobility and sleep.*

• *Glucosamine, Chondroitin & MSM: are essential sulfates to help with joint pain, bone repair, arthritis, and osteoarthritis. This combo helps heal and restore cartilage and bones (in caps, liquids, shots).*

• *Herbs for Healthy Bones: here are many herbs to help improve circulation and bone strength. Herbs help heal broken bones and relieve tendon and joint pain. List of healing herbs include:*

Wild Yam Root, Horsetail Herb, Oatstraw, Sarsaparilla Root, White Oak Bark, Comfrey, Marshmallow, Alfalfa, Black Cohash, Barley Grass, Garlic, Plantain, Propolis, Goldenseal, Silica, Dandelion, Nettles, Arnica, Kelp, Sea Greens. At health stores in powder form, caps, tinctures and teas. – Linda Page, N.D., Ph.D., healthyhealing.com

Collagen Promotes Healthy Bones, Skin and Ligaments

The organic matter in our bones consists mainly of collagen, the "glue" that holds together our skin, tendons, ligaments and bones. Zinc, copper, beta-carotene, sulfur, L-lysine, proline and vitamin C are important in helping promote and maintain healthy collagen in the body.

Eat Plenty of Cabbage – The Miracle Cleanser and Healer

Cabbage (raw) has amazing properties. It stimulates the immune system, kills bacteria and viruses, heals ulcers, and according to Dr. James Balch in Prescription for Cooking and Dietary Wellness, *your chances of contracting colon cancer can be reduced by up to 60% by eating cabbage weekly. Dr. Saxon-Graham states that those who never consumed cabbage were three times more likely to develop colon cancer. A Japanese study shows that people who ate cabbage had the lowest fatality rate from any cancer. Therapeutic benefits have also been attributed to cabbage in relation to scurvy, gout, rheumatism (arthritis), eye diseases, asthma, pyorrhea, and gangrene. See our Bragg Salad Recipe (page 79). Cooking destroys the cabbages healing properties. We love cabbage and also we make a variety of sandwiches wrapped in cabbage leaves instead of bread. Try this – so delicious!!!*

3. Massage and Physiotherapy: Many forms of massage and physiotherapy can increase vital circulation to help nourish your cartilage, connective tissues and to break up unhealthy, painful deposits in your joints and tissues. There are many therapies to choose from in Chapter 11 under Alternative Therapies (pages 117 to 120).

4. Exercise and Movement: Commonly, those who are already experiencing pain are advised to rest, and this feels appropriate because pain usually means *stop!* However, studies show that continued activity in spite of pain actually can lessen pain through release of endorphins and strengthen joints as well. Ice and anti-inflammatory creams, DMSO (pat on), etc., (*see page 91*) can be used to help lessen discomfort. Hydro (water, hot & cold) therapy also makes easier, pain-free gentle movement possible for many. Regular practice of gentle Yoga, Pilates, Anderson and Bragg stretching exercises also helps maintain healthy flexibility, range of motion and reduces stiffness. Remember what the Greeks knew and practiced over 5,000 years ago – moderation in all things! The last thing you want to do is overextend yourself and make the problem worse. That's why it's important to keep in close contact with your chiropractor and other health care providers.

According to Dr. John Bland, professor of medicine at the University of Vermont and one of the country's leading arthritis experts, the most common form of arthritis and osteoarthritis, occurs because of dysfunction of the molecules of connective tissue that line the surface of a joint. These collagen molecules can become frayed and irritated by overuse due to obesity, basic disuse, or misapplied pressure from an injury or congenitally misaligned joint. A carefully moderated exercise plan, plus diet helps keep weight down and increases muscular strength, flexibility and endurance in order to protect all your various body joints from these unhealthy pressures.

19

Websites to check for Herbal Remedies:
• healthydirections.com • healthyhealing.com • kcweb.com/herb

To preserve health is a moral and religious duty, for health is the basis for all social virtues. We can't be as useful when not well.
– Dr. Samuel Johnson, Father of Dictionaries

In Rare Cases, Prevention May Be Too Late

In extremely advanced cases of joint deterioration, sometimes the only option is surgery. There has been a good deal of success with these procedures, and research is advancing the practice almost constantly.

The first kind of surgery is called osteotomy, in which damaged bone and tissue are removed and the joint is restored to its proper position.

Next are joint replacement surgeries, which can be either partial or complete, cemented or uncemented. Your board certified orthopedist can help you to determine which is best for you, and we always recommend that you get at least three opinions before committing to any invasive surgery. The following illustrations show what is involved in total joint replacements.

One amazing new development that has advanced hip replacement surgery is a new computer, the Medmodeler, that can make three-dimensional, plastic models of a patient's exact bone structure. According to Douglas Robertson, M.D., Washington University School of Medicine (who created the machine), *"There's something about holding models in your hand. They have the tactile sense surgeons need."*
• *Is the prosthesis tight?* • *Does it rub?* • *What size really fits?*

Total Joint Replacements

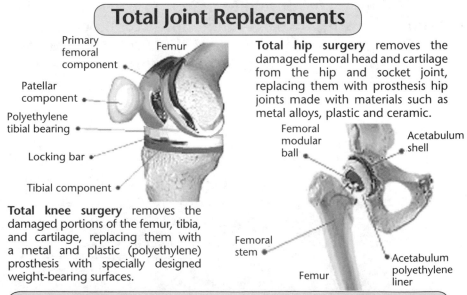

Primary femoral component

Femur

Patellar component

Polyethylene tibial bearing

Locking bar

Tibial component

Total hip surgery removes the damaged femoral head and cartilage from the hip and socket joint, replacing them with prosthesis hip joints made with materials such as metal alloys, plastic and ceramic.

Femoral modular ball

Acetabulum shell

Femoral stem

Femur

Acetabulum polyethylene liner

Total knee surgery removes the damaged portions of the femur, tibia, and cartilage, replacing them with a metal and plastic (polyethylene) prosthesis with specially designed weight-bearing surfaces.

Check out website: www.jointreplacement.com

Composition of the Bones

To be healthy and strong, both cartilage and bones need a full daily ration of organic calcium, phosphorus, magnesium and manganese (natural sources of these minerals will be given in a later section on nutrition).

The long bones, such as the arms and legs, are generally cylindrical in shape, and the long portion is called the shaft. The ends of these bones are thicker and are shaped to fit into the ends of the adjoining bones to form the various types of joints described in the preceding section. The short bones, such as those of the wrist and ankle, are composed mostly of a thick shaft of elastic, spongy material inside a thin covering of hard bone material. Flat bones, such as the ribs, are made up of spongy material between plates of hard bone.

A cross section of the bone shows the two main types of material of which it is composed. The *hard outer material* that gives bone its shape and strength consists primarily of chemical compounds of calcium and phosphorus. The bones and teeth contain 90% of the body's calcium. This is why calcium is required more than any other mineral for body tissue repair.

The *soft inner part* of the bone is called marrow. Most bone marrow is yellowish in color, made up of fat cells and serving as a storage depot for fat which can be converted into energy as the body's needs require. Toward the ends of the long bones and generally throughout the interior of the flat bones (such as those of the skull and the spinal column), patches and streaks of reddish tissue show in the marrow. These are the vital manufacturing centers of the red blood cells (or corpuscles), which transport life-giving oxygen throughout the body. The white blood corpuscles, which combat infection, are also produced in the bone marrow.

A teacher for the day can be a guiding light for a lifetime!
Bragg Books are silent health teachers – never tiring, ready night or day to help you help yourself to health and are your friends for life! Our books are written with love and we have a deep desire to guide you to a healthy lifestyle for a long, healthy, happy fulfilled life. – Patricia Bragg

Bones Help Protect Your Vital Organs

Bones also protect the softer parts of the body, especially vital organs. The skull forms a strong case for the soft gray matter of the brain. Two bony sockets in front of the skull protect the eyes. The spinal column is a bony tube that safeguards the delicate, vital spinal cord.

The ribs form a hard, elastic framework that protects the heart and lungs. If a person had no ribs and bumped into something, even a small bump might collapse the lungs or damage the heart. The lower rib cage also shelters, in the back and at the sides, and the kidneys and major organs of the upper digestive system. The important protecting ribs are supported by the spinal column.

The pelvic bones, which include the base of the spinal column (sacrum and coccyx) and the hip bones, protect the bladder and the reproductive organs.

Structure of the Spinal Column

How is this marvelous pivot of the human skeleton constructed? To illustrate some of its functions, we have likened it to the ridgepole of a house or the main pole of a tent. The spine is not a single rigid bone; if it was, the motions of the human body would be very limited. The spine is a flexible column composed of 26 bones: 24 small vertebrae from the base of the skull to the pelvic region, the sacrum (which is actually the natural fusion of five embryonic vertebrae into a wedge-shaped bone that forms the back of the pelvis) and the coccyx (or tail bone, the small triangular bone of four fused embryonic vertebrae at the base of the sacrum). During its growth inside the womb, a human embryo first develops 33 vertebrae; the lower nine fuse into the sacrum and coccyx before birth.

At birth, the human spine forms a single, arched curve. As the baby begins to lift his head and sit erect, the seven upper vertebrae between the base of the skull and the shoulders (forming neck) strengthen into what is known as the cervical curve. The ribs are attached at back of chest, at the next 12 vertebrae, known as thoracic vertebrae, larger than cervical vertebrae for more heavier work support.

A healthy flexible spine leads to a healthy life!

Central Nervous System & Spine

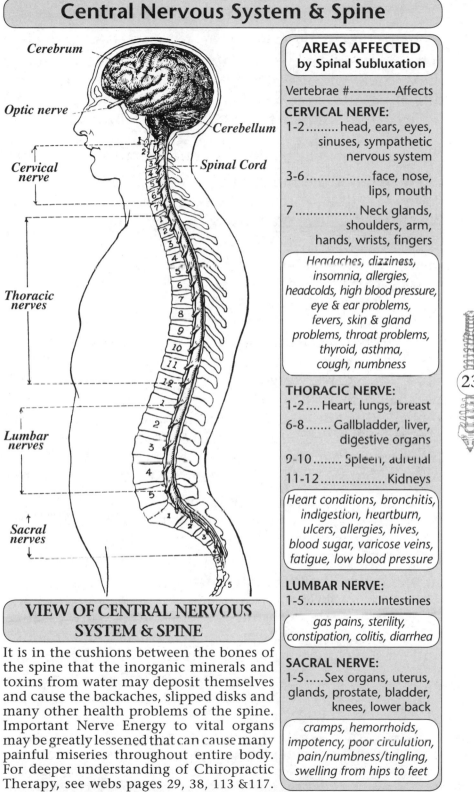

Cerebrum

Optic nerve

Cerebellum

Spinal Cord

Cervical nerve

Thoracic nerves

Lumbar nerves

Sacral nerves

VIEW OF CENTRAL NERVOUS SYSTEM & SPINE

It is in the cushions between the bones of the spine that the inorganic minerals and toxins from water may deposit themselves and cause the backaches, slipped disks and many other health problems of the spine. Important Nerve Energy to vital organs may be greatly lessened that can cause many painful miseries throughout entire body. For deeper understanding of Chiropractic Therapy, see webs pages 29, 38, 113 &117.

AREAS AFFECTED
by Spinal Subluxation

Vertebrae #----------Affects

CERVICAL NERVE:

1-2 .... head, ears, eyes, sinuses, sympathetic nervous system

3-6 .... face, nose, lips, mouth

7 .... Neck glands, shoulders, arm, hands, wrists, fingers

Headaches, dizziness, insomnia, allergies, headcolds, high blood pressure, eye & ear problems, fevers, skin & gland problems, throat problems, thyroid, asthma, cough, numbness

THORACIC NERVE:

1-2 .... Heart, lungs, breast

6-8 .... Gallbladder, liver, digestive organs

9-10 .... Spleen, adrenal

11-12 .... Kidneys

Heart conditions, bronchitis, indigestion, heartburn, ulcers, allergies, hives, blood sugar, varicose veins, fatigue, low blood pressure

LUMBAR NERVE:

1-5 .... Intestines

gas pains, sterility, constipation, colitis, diarrhea

SACRAL NERVE:

1-5 ..... Sex organs, uterus, glands, prostate, bladder, knees, lower back

cramps, hemorrhoids, impotency, poor circulation, pain/numbness/tingling, swelling from hips to feet

23

Early Development of the Spine

When the baby begins to stand erect and walk, the next five vertebrae adjust to form the inward lumbar curve (small of back). The sacrum curves backward again, attaching at sacroiliac joints to the hip bones, and the little coccyx completes the spine with an inward turn.

These natural, shallow S-curves of the spinal column are the bases of the resilient strength that makes it the mainspring of the human body. The components of this spring are the vertebrae. The vertebrae are intricately constructed, in two main parts: the body and spinal arch.

The round body of the vertebra projects inward, a solid piece of spongily textured bone that forms the weight-bearing part of the spinal column. The top and bottom of each vertebral body is covered with a thin, circular plate of cartilage. Between the bodies of each two vertebrae is a cushioning intervertebral disk, a marvelous little mechanism composed of a thin, elastic outside covering of fibrocartilage, with a semifluidic center. These disks, which we shall discuss later in more detail, make it possible for the spinal column to move comfortably in many various directions, from bending and stretching to absorbing shocks. If it were not for these disks, you would feel a blow at the base of your skull every time you sat down or took a step.

The spinal arches of the vertebrae form the opening, or canal, for passage and protection of the spinal cord. At back of each arch are five fingerlike bony projections, to which the intricate system of back ligaments and muscles are anchored. The central projections, known as spinous processes, are what you feel as your *backbone* (like a train track). Joining each vertebra are gliding, interlocking joints that project vertically from each arch and are enveloped by capsules lined with synovial fluid.

The miracle human body has one ability not possessed by any machine – the ability to repair and heal itself. – George E. Crile, Jr., M.D.

"Your arteries are living structures with vital functions. Their linings have about 98 different enzymatic systems, whose purpose is not only to prevent blockage damage, but to allow oxygen and nutrients to permeate freely through them into the heart muscles and other tissues." – Dr. Savely Yurkovsky, Cardiologist

The Spine and the Muscular System

Although the intervertebral joints add flexibility and sturdiness to the spine, what really holds the spinal column together and in shape are the strong, tough ligaments that weave in and out of the finger projections of the spinal arches. Extending from the skull to the sacrum, these powerful, elastic ligaments lace together all the vertebrae and intervertebral disks. Another system of extremely tough ligaments is woven back and forth throughout the sacroiliac area to give the tremendous support necessary to hold together these joints between hips and spine base (which bears most body's weight and obesity overburdens).

The Muscles of the Human Body

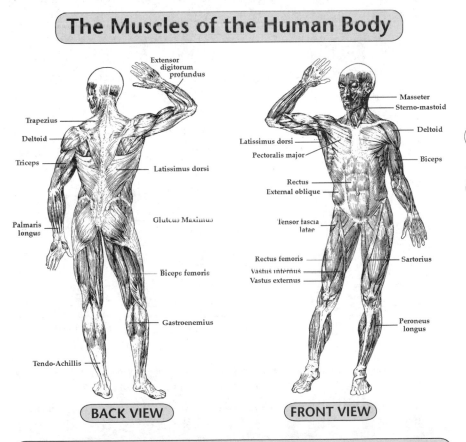

Extensor digitorum profundus

Trapezius
Deltoid
Triceps
Latissimus dorsi
Palmaris longus
Gluteus Maximus
Biceps femoris
Gastroenemius
Tendo-Achillis

BACK VIEW

Masseter
Sterno-mastoid
Deltoid
Latissimus dorsi
Pectoralis major
Biceps
Rectus
External oblique
Tensor fascia latae
Rectus femoris
Vastus internus
Vastus externus
Sartorius
Peroneus longus

FRONT VIEW

25

There are over 640 muscles in the body. All physical body functions involve muscle activity. These functions include skeletal movements, contraction of the heart, in the gut and many more. Three different types of muscles are responsible for these activities: skeletal muscles, cardiac muscles and smooth muscles, all of these important muscles have some characteristics in common.

Spine Motion Exercises Promote Spine Health

An elaborate system of muscles is also attached to the vertebrae by tendons to hold the vertebrae in place when the body is at rest, yet allow them to move when the body is in motion. These muscles and the interwoven ligaments around the spinal column are what the Spine Motion Exercises are designed to activate. These exercises are especially designed to achieve and maintain full length and flexibility of the spinal column.

Without muscles to operate the levers, sockets, pivots and gliders of the skeletal system, our skeletons would remain a mere assemblage of static bones. Just as it is the pivot of the skeletal system, the spinal column is the anchor point of the muscular system! Layers of powerful back and abdomen muscles manipulate the body's major movements: bending forward, backward and sideways; reaching upward; lifting; carrying; pulling and pushing. Movements of the head and neck are accomplished by muscles anchored to upper cervical vertebrae. Shoulder and upper-arm muscles anchor to cervical, thoracic and upper lumbar vertebrae, while thigh muscles anchor to the sacrum and coccyx. The muscles operating in our breathing apparatus are anchored to the spine: the diaphragm to lumbar vertebrae and rib muscles to thoracocervical vertebrae. Pelvic muscles, supporting the viscera and important for good elimination, are anchored to the lower spine.

The Spine "Shrinks" and Ages With Disuse

Even with the operation of all these muscles, the daily activities of the average person does not fully exercise the spine. Its built-in capacity is seldom if ever used, especially in today's under-exercised, malnourished affluent society. We are a civilization of sitters and spectator sportsmen, overfed and malnourished by devitalized, artificial foods.

No wonder back pain is the second most common cause of missed work days, and leading cause of disability between active ages of 19 to 60, and the number one impairment in occupational injuries. An estimated eight out of ten people have back problems some time in their life. Please – You don't have to be one of these people!

No man can violate Nature's Laws and escape her penalties. – Julian Johnson

Exercise & Healthy Foods Make Strong Bones

The overall health condition of your spine can determine how fast it will recover from pain and risk of a condition becoming chronic. Muscles become flabby from lack of regular exercise and tissues depleted from lack of proper nourishment. Unused and misused, the spine then *settles,* stiffens and often becomes visibly misshapen. Dependent on exercise and good circulation in adjacent tissues for their nourishment, cartilage and disks between the vertebrae start deteriorating. The unstretched spinal column *shrinks and ages!* Many people in their 60s and 70s become up to three to five inches shorter in height, often called *bent over by old age.*

It is not age, however, that causes the spine to shorten or become bent into abnormal curvature. Deficiency in diet and insufficient or incorrect exercise are so prevalent that many American children and adolescents scuff along with slumped spines, poor posture and no energy. The longer this condition persists, the more pronounced it becomes. That is why it is attributed to age.

If time were the only factor, my Dad's spine would be fossilized, as a man with grown great, great-grandchildren; yet, his spine is just as long, flexible and just as strong as it was more than 60 years ago. Why? Because he knows the vital importance of exercising the spinal column to keep good circulation in his spinal region and of maintaining the muscles and ligaments that hold the spine in place in top tone and fitness. Plus, Dad and I know the essential value of eating natural healthy organic foods that contain the important minerals and vitamins to build strong, healthy bones and cartilage! No spine is any stronger than the food material of which it is made, and no spine is any stronger than the exercise it is given, regardless of your calendar years. Nothing affects your entire life, health, energy and vitality as much as the condition of your spinal column.

It was Confucius who said: "Eat not for the pleasure thou mayest find therein; eat to increase thy strength and health, eat to preserve the life thou has received from Heaven!"

You Can Have a Youthful Spine at Any Age, says Paul C. Bragg

Bernarr Macfadden, Physical Culture's founding father, was my mentor and gave me my start in health crusading and writing. Macfadden often said: *You are as young as your spine. Any man or woman can take twenty to thirty years off their age by just straightening and stretching up their spine with good posture. It's literally so. It's been done, and is being done. You can prevent the process called ageing or repair its inroads on your health to an amazing extent by Spine Motion Exercises and proper nutrition. When gently extended to elastic capacity, nothing in physiology acts as quickly and positively as the spinal column.*

Consider the fact that almost all people usually feel their best in the morning upon rising. This is not only due to a refreshing sleep, but also because the spine has lengthened by its long rest. You have often heard that you are taller in the morning; in truth, you are. (*You can verify this by doing comparative measurements.*) The longer length brought about by repose is very quickly lost, as the upright position and activities of the day cause the spine once again to settle unless you have strengthened the spinal column and its supporting ligaments and muscles by a systematic program of exercise, posture and nutrition (*as given in this book*). Very few people exercise the spine sufficiently, and the cartilage (*protective cushions between bones*) and disks become *squeezed*. Subjected to constant friction between the vertebrae, cartilage can wear thin and cause painful complications. The disks are subject to degenerative changes such as calcification. As a result, not only do the bony surfaces of the vertebrae rub against each other, but they also impinge on, or *pinch*, the nerves from the spinal cord through vertebral openings, causing uncomfortable, nagging pain

28

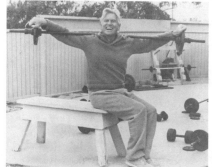

It has been proven in a Boston University Study, done by Dr. Maria A. Fiatarone, that weight-lifting improves overall health, especially back health. A frail group of nursing home residents, ages 75-96, were given a high intensity weight lifting program. At the end of 8 weeks they had stronger, more youthful backs. Paul and Patricia lift weights 3 times weekly.
See www.jcaaa.org/liftingweights.htm

Spine Motion Helps Keep Spine Youthful

Miraculously, the cartilage responds readily to the stimulation of these Spine Motion Exercises, which are designed to stretch the spinal column and open the natural spacing between the vertebrae. Cartilage grows from the moment it's given room to develop. It's this quick restoration of cartilage (plus nutrition) that makes it so astonishingly easy to accomplish apparent wonders with Spine Motion Exercises, irrespective of the person's age. In fact, age effects cartilage growth less than almost any form of replacement in the body. It's possible to produce abundant cartilage, and to have a biologically youthful spine, regardless of your calendar years!

What Is a "Slipped Disk"?

The chief shock absorbers of the spinal column and the *ball bearings* that give it such great flexibility and resilience are the intervertebral disks. These little cushions between the vertebrae are composed of a *stuffing* of extremely elastic tissue. The tissue is the consistency of a pudding but very tough, called the nucleus pulposus, which is encased in a laminated (layered) covering called the annulus, resembling an onion but exceptionally tough and resilient. It is reinforced at the top and bottom by the cartilage plates, which protect the disk from contact with the bone.

29

When the spine flexes, in whatever direction, the disks are compressed in that direction, pushing the nucleus in the opposite direction to fill the extra space there between the vertebrae. In strong, healthy spines, the *ball bearing* function of these disks can withstand a great deal of pressure. However, if the annulus (covering) becomes weakened, or if the disk is subjected to severe compression by a sudden accident, jolt or undue strain, the pressure on the nucleus pushes it through the outer covering into the spinal canal. In medical terms, this is called a ruptured intervertebral disk, disc, or herniated nucleus pulposus (known as a *slipped disk*). When this occurs, the disk is pushed (*slipped*) out into the spinal canal.

Exercise is important for overall health and should not be avoided. Low-impact activities such as swimming, walking and bicycling (winter use stationary bicycle) can increase overall fitness without straining the lower back. – www.webmd.com

Slipped Disc blocks passageway and produces damaging pressure on the spinal cord. At the same time, the adjoining vertebrae, robbed of their cushion, then press against each other and on the nerves coming out from the spinal cord. Until this injury became so prevalent during World War II, primarily from bouncing in jeeps over rugged terrain, the resulting severe pain was frequently diagnosed as sciatica or other known forms of lower back pain. Once the true cause was discovered, however, remedial surgical techniques were developed. These have now become so perfected, as well as methods of diagnosis, that practically normal spinal function can be restored. In addition to avoiding sudden or severe strains, the best way to avoid a future slipped disk is to lengthen and strengthen up your spine with our Spine Motion Exercises, good posture and healthy nourishment, so that your disks will be strong, healthy, tough and resilient.

Alternatives to Painful Back Surgery

Our 23 spinal disks help give our spine its sideways curves (a curved spine is sixteen times stronger than a straight one) and also join the vertebrae together. Disks contribute to our height – in the morning we are about $1/4$" – $1/2$" taller than we were the night before because our disks thin a little during the day and expand a little while we sleep. The disks themselves don't actually *slip*, since they are knitted into the vertebrae from above and below. What sometimes do slip are the vertebrae, which may put pressure on the disk and contribute to its damage. Many *slipped disks* would be more accurately called *slipped vertebrae*. Since regular x-rays cannot *see* a disk, the MRI or CT scans are necessary to reveal any disk problems. In some instances the EMG (electromyography) is also of great value, as this will show the nerves and muscles also. Ironically, it is not unusual to find people with no pain show herniation, even ruptured disks, while others with pain show no disk problems at all. This demonstrates the complexities of spinal pain.

Heat treatment gives good results for chronic back pain. A nonsurgical procedure called Intradiscal Electrothermal Therapy (IDET) provides lasting improvements for patients with chronic-disc related back pain that do not respond to conventional back treatments reports the journal Spine. The heat toughens and seals the disc, as well as destroying any abnormal nerve endings. See webs: www.idet-spinetherapy.com and www.spine.org

> **Nobody should have back surgery unless they have seen a chiropractor first.** – Robert Mendelsohn, M.D

The medical approach to disk problems is often a combination of painkillers, muscle relaxers, and physical therapy. It may involve hot or cold packs, baths, traction, electrical stimulation, and as a last resort, surgery.

The first steps to deal with herniated disk problems are conservative. These include rest, analgesics, chiropractic and physical therapy. At this point it's convenient to have X-rays done in search of indirect evidence of the disk problem, and see if any degenerative changes exist on the spine. If these measures fail, the possibility of surgery may be contemplated, based on examinations using MRI (magnetic resonance imaging) or CT (computer tomography) to show the disk, any rupture, etc., and the space behind it and the nerves. The EMG (electromyography) shows nerves and muscles.

If you do suffer from a slipped/herniated/ruptured disk, consider a more natural alternative before you consider drastic surgery. There are over 600,000 back surgeries performed per year with an average failure rate of 53%. Non-operative approaches can have a 96% success rate, and Cauda Equina Syndrome, which includes buttock numbness, leg weakness, and bladder and bowel disfunction, is the only absolute indication for surgery. There are some surgical treatments receiving praise, like the endoscopic processes performed by board certified neuro or orthopedic surgeons, that do help in some cases. After any surgery, of course, the complete recovery program is important: proper exercise, sound diet, proper rest and entire body health maintenance.

If you must resort to surgery, microdisectomy takes an hour on outpatient basis. As opposed to more serious surgery methods. Skin openings made are just large enough to admit scope and remove a millimeter of bone above or below herniated/ruptured disk without altering spine structure. Usually occurs at levels L4-L5 or L5-S1. Only specially trained board certified orthopedic or neuro-surgeons are best for this procedure (*www.backinstitute.com*).

Alternative For Healing Slipped Disk

A non-invasive alternative is the VAX-D® or Vertebral Axial Decompression introduced in 1991 by Allen E. Dyer, M.D. It carefully stretches and relaxes spine in cycles and has good success rate. Patient is fitted with patented pelvic harness designed to carefully stretch lumbar spine. VAX-D® device then applies precisely controlled tension along axis of spinal column to distract vertebral segments and rear-facing facets of lumbar spine, thus decompressing intervertebral disks. Each distraction cycle, lasting 60 seconds, is followed by relaxation cycle of similar duration. Sessions include about 15 of these cycles and last about 30 minutes, and the number and precise nature of sessions varies with individual patient. The treatment is effective, safe and cost-effective without the risks associated with drugs, surgery or injections. Clinical studies have found this simple method to be successful in over 70% of patients. It provides early return to work without any hospitalization. (See web: *www.vaxd.com*)

Take Whiplash Injuries to Your Chiropractor

Chiropractic, in contrast to most other treatments, has done well over the years helping prevent many whiplash injuries from becoming painful and chronic. Because of their high success record with treating whiplash injuries, researchers worldwide are now studying chiropractic treatment methods. We have seen miracles and have benefitted ourselves when needed.

Recently a group of medical researchers from Dublin, Ireland compared a treatment approach similar to that used by chiropractors with that of medication and rest. Sixty-one patients seen at the emergency room for whiplash injury were divided into two groups to receive these two different treatments. The group receiving manipulation had the greater reduction of pain and return of movement than did the group treated with medication, rest and neck collars. These results led the researchers to conclude that whiplash is better treated with early active chiropractic treatment. Many people suffering from whiplash injury could avoid prolonged or permanent suffering by receiving chiropractic care the medical researchers discovered.

Physiotherapy & Chiropractic should be used in treating whiplash.

Chapter 3

Your Precious Nerve Force

Spinal Cord: the Body's Vital "Control Center"

The most important function of the spine is to protect the spinal cord, the vital *control center* without which the musculoskeletal system and other vital organs of the body could not operate. Not even the most sophisticated computer system can match the performance of this cord of nerve tissue. Less than 12 feet long, little more than 3-inch in diameter and weighing about an ounce . . .

> the spinal cord is the calculator and relay center of a vast and intricate miracle network of nerves that reach into every part of the human body.

The spinal cord passes through the canal formed by the vertebral arches, continuous with and extending downward from the base of the brain (*medulla oblongata*). At the first lumbar vertebra, the single cord ends in a number of delicate filaments or threads that extend to the end of the spine and fasten the spinal cord to the coccyx. Cerebrospinal fluid maintains pressure in the cord, which is insulated from the bony canal by three layers of coverings called meninges.

THE NERVOUS SYSTEM IS THE COMMUNICATION SYSTEM OF YOUR BODY

Your nervous system is made up of vital nerves which extend throughout your body and brain and vary noticeably in diameter.

33

Men do not die, they kill themselves with wrong habits.
– Seneca, Roman Philosopher

Spinal Nerves Control Our Actions

The spinal nerves pass through openings in the vertebral arches and branch out to serve various parts of the body. There are 31 pairs of these nerves: 8 cervical, 12 thoracic, five lumbar, five sacral and one coccygeal. Roots of the sensory nerves, which convey feeling, are attached to the back or dorsal side of the spinal cord. Roots of the corresponding motor nerves, controlling action, are attached to the front or ventral side. Each pair controls a specific part of the body. Example: if you stub your toe against a piece of furniture, the branch of the sensory nerve to that leg and foot flashes a pain signal to the central control in the spinal cord, and the matching motor nerve immediately transmits the order to pull back your foot. This is done so swiftly that your reaction seems instantaneous.

Except for those controlled by the 12 cranial (brain) nerves, automatic or reflex actions are controlled by the spinal cord. For example, we *see* in our brain via the cranial optic nerve, but certain eye muscles are controlled from the spinal cord, and we *cry* by order of a spinal nerve that controls the lachrymal gland. Conscious actions naturally originate in the brain, but when these become reflex, they are usually transferred to the control center of the spinal cord.

In computer terminology, the brain *programs* a course of action and when it becomes habit it becomes part of the *database* of the spinal cord. When you learn to drive a car, for example, at first you must consciously think out every move, but with practice, it becomes automatic. Experienced drivers automatically calculate the speed of their own and other cars on the road, then decide how much acceleration will be required to pass safely. If they had to stop and figure this out consciously, they would never pass another car; but it is done in a split-second by their spinal nerve reflexes. The same sort of thing happens in emergencies and in countless daily actions (such as walking, sitting, eating, talking, etc.) programmed from infancy. Already in the database of our spinal miracle computer at birth is its lifelong role in regulating our breathing, heartbeat, circulation, digestion, elimination and reproductive functions, your a miracle!

The Autonomic Nervous System Your Spinal Database Computer

Here are the two divisions: the Craniosacral or Parasympathetic, and the Thoracolumbar or Sympathetic.

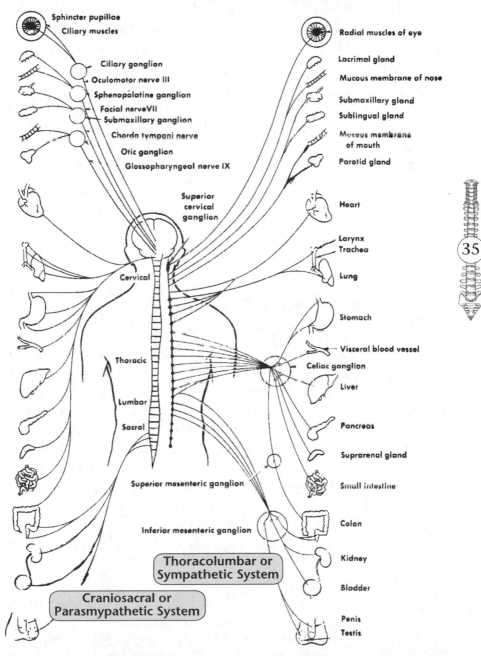

Sphincter pupillae
Ciliary muscles

Ciliary ganglion
Oculomotor nerve III
Sphenopalatine ganglion
Facial nerve VII
Submaxillary ganglion
Chorda tympani nerve
Otic ganglion
Glossopharyngeal nerve IX

Superior cervical ganglion

Cervical

Thoracic

Lumbar

Sacral

Superior mesenteric ganglion

Inferior mesenteric ganglion

Radial muscles of eye
Lacrimal gland
Mucous membrane of nose
Submaxillary gland
Sublingual gland
Mucous membrane of mouth
Parotid gland
Heart
Larynx
Trachea
Lung
Stomach
Visceral blood vessel
Celiac ganglion
Liver
Pancreas
Suprarenal gland
Small intestine
Colon
Kidney
Bladder
Penis
Testis

Thoracolumbar or Sympathetic System

Craniosacral or Parasmypathetic System

The Spine and Nervous System

Now you see why it's so important to keep your spine long, strong and flexible. It is made to protect your spinal cord and to stay in perfect alignment while also allowing freedom of flexible body movements in all directions.

Through our nerves we experience every physical pleasure or pain. The spine, when kept straight, strong, flexible and elongated, allows every set of nerves to function freely. The spine that has settled or shortened has less space between the vertebrae, crowding the nerves that pass through openings in the vertebral arches. This finally causes painful pressure on the bones and the nerves.

When such impingement occurs in the upper cervical vertebrae, at the base of the head or upper neck, it may bring on headaches. Occurring an inch farther down, the eye muscles may be strained. In the thoracic area, pressure on nerves to the stomach and/or other digestive organs may cause malfunction or distress there. Farther down, impingement may affect bowels or kidneys. In fact, there's no body part that is not affected in some way by the spinal nervous system, as page 23 chart and graphics show.

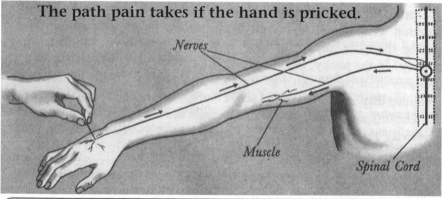

The path pain takes if the hand is pricked.

Nerves

Muscle

Spinal Cord

Good Posture – Good for Your Health

Poor posture distorts the alignment of bones, chronically tenses muscles, and contributes to stressful conditions such as: loss of vital lung capacity, increased fatigue, reduced blood and oxygen to the brain, limited range of motion, stiffness of joints, pain syndromes, reduced mental alertness, and decreased productivity at work.

The more mechanically out of alignment a person is, the less energy is available for thinking, metabolism & healing. – Dr. Roger Sperry, Nobel Laureate

POSTURE SILHOUETTES: Which one are you?

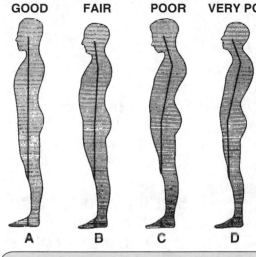

GOOD   **FAIR**   **POOR**   **VERY POOR**

A B C D

A Good: Head, trunk and thigh in a straight line; chest high and forward; abdomen flat; back curves normally.

B Fair: Head too forward; abdomen too prominent; exaggerated curve in upper back; slightly hollow lower back.

C Poor: Relaxed posture; head too forward; abdomen relaxed; shoulder blades prominent; hollow lower back.

D Very Poor: Head too far forward; very exaggerated curve in upper back; abdomen relaxed; chest flat-sloping;

Back, Vertebrae and Spine Injuries

When an accident or injury even slightly displaces a vertebra, the acute pain causes the victim immediately to seek out expert treatment. When the displacement occurs gradually, however, the warning pain is often erroneously attributed to the affected organ or area of the body, rather than the cause of a misalignment, strain, pinched spinal nerve, etc. The difference is only in degree. A dislocation, an obvious, violent disarrangement through injury or strain, when sudden, is felt acutely. The settling process by which a vertebra becomes improperly positioned is often gradual; it may even begin to grow that way during teenage years.

The slow erosion of cartilage and weakening of muscles and ligaments may go unnoticed, because of the body's amazing natural ability to compensate and the built-in power of the spine to withstand punishment. When vertebraes come so close together that they impoverish any set of nerves, some part of the human mechanism slows down, weakens, suffers and draws unduly on nervous vitality in an effort to overcome the handicap. This causes back pain for millions.

Good posture helps prevent backaches and related problems.

Staying in shape pays, partly because aerobic activity promotes circulation. If you already have back problems, the right kind of regular exercise will help prevent you from getting more severe pain and further injury. – Stephen Hochschuler, M.D., Chairman of the Texas Back Institute in Plano, Texas • www.texasback.com

Nerve Energy is Essential to Health

Nerve energy is so essential to mental and physical health that we recommend you read more about it in our companion text, *Building Powerful Nerve Force*.

Here, we are primarily concerned with the spinal column and its relationship to the part of the central nervous system that is controlled by the spinal cord. For peak performance of these nerves, which greatly influence the health of your entire body, a fully flexible, strong, healthy, elongated spine is vitally essential. We believe in prevention. Your friendly chiropractor is interested in helping you maintain a healthy spine and body! It's wise to have your spine checked from time to time by your chiropractor, who will help you with his specialized knowledge and training in displaced vertebrae and back and neck problems. Your chiropractor will help you keep your spine strong, healthy and in perfect alignment, if you will do your part and keep the muscles strong and healthy by doing these Spine Motion Exercises.

38

See these websites on Chiropractic Therapy:
• *www.chiropractic.org* • *www.chiroweb.com/find* • *www.hqchiro.com*

A healthy, flexible, aligned spine goes a long way in helping you stay youthful for a long, healthy life! – Shawn Miller, D.C., perfecthealthnow.com

Adequate healthy food is the cradle of normal resistance, the playground of normal immunity, the workshop of good health, and the laboratory of long life.
– Dr. Charles Mayo, founder of the famous Mayo Clinic

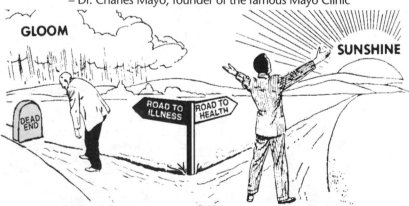

GLOOM

SUNSHINE

DEAD END

ROAD TO ILLNESS

ROAD TO HEALTH

NEGATIVE ⇦ OR ⇨ POSITIVE
The choice of which road to take is up to you.
You alone decide whether to reach a dead end or live a healthy lifestyle for a long, healthy, happy, active life. – Paul C. Bragg

Chapter 4

Doctor Posture Works Miracles

Proper Posture is Continuous Exercise

Before we go into the special Spine Motion Exercises, we must establish the basic exercise, which should be so thoroughly programmed into your nervous system that you practice it all the time: standing, sitting, walking, lying down. This continuous exercise is the habit of proper posture. It begins in infancy and continues throughout life.

Posture means how we hold our bodies. Proper posture is the balanced alignment of the body. When standing erect, an imaginary plumb line representing the center of gravity should fall in alignment with the top center of the skull through the center of the ear, and through the centers of the joints at the shoulder, to the rest of the body; shoulders straight; chest up and not in an exaggerated stance; keep abdomen firm and lift up chest

39

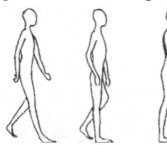

Walking Posture:

Walking posture: Always prepare a new base before leaving the old.

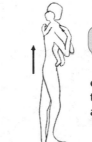

Lifting Posture:

Lifting weight: The weight of the baby is held close to the center of gravity directly above the pushing force.

Standing posture is important – your ears, shoulders, hips and knees should be in line with one another.

Good posture is a way of doing things with more energy, less stress and fatigue. Without good posture, you cannot really be physically fit. – www.hqchiro.com

off waist. In this position, the spine holds its natural, gentle curves, and weight of the body is supported by the hips and feet, slightly apart, with stress on the heels.

To sum it up, *Stand tall!* To get that tall feeling, imagine that a powerful giant is holding you by the hair and almost lifting you off the ground. You should not only stand tall, you must also sit tall and walk tall. If you have been slouching or slumping, as most people do, you will probably find that this erect posture is uncomfortable at first, because your muscles and ligaments have become too slack or too tense from being held in the wrong positions and not properly exercised.

Let Your Mirror Be Your Judge

To find out literally *the true shape you're in,* stand in front of a full-length mirror and critically view yourself as you would a stranger. Examine your front. Using the reflection from a hand mirror, examine your sides and then your back. Wear only a swimsuit, or nothing at all! Let your mirror mercilessly reveal the truth.

Does your head stick forward? Do your shoulders slump? Is one shoulder or hip higher than the other? Is your upper back round? Do you have a pot belly? Are you swayback? Does your spine curve to one side?

Analyze your posture defects (pg. 44), list them by date on a chart. Keep a weekly record of your progress toward perfect posture, reexamining yourself mercilessly in the mirror each week as you carry out this Fitness Program with Spine Motion Exercises. If you faithfully follow the instructions in this book, you will be highly gratified by the results, in both health and a more youthful appearance and well-being.

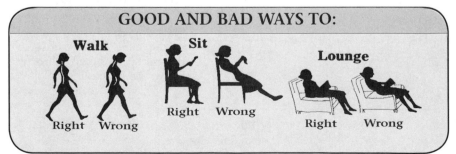

Improve your posture – it is critically important to improving how you feel.

Bragg Posture Exercise
Promotes Health and Youthfulness

Here's a simple way to check and reset your posture every day. Stand tall with your feet a comfortable ten inches apart and your toes pointing straight forward. Put your hands on buttocks and tighten buttocks. Move hands to lower stomach muscles and suck in stomach muscles. Move hands up to lower rib cage, stretch up spine and lift rib cage up. Move hands to upper chest; lift chest up. Move hands to shoulders; lift them up and slightly back. Put right hand under chin and lift chin up. Now line body up straight, nose plumb-line to belly button, and drop hands heavy to sides, swinging them easily back and forth. This normalizes posture naturally and helps you find the posture best for you. Look in the mirror to see if the shoulders are level. You may have to lift one shoulder up a little to equalize and level them. Usually, with practice, they will become naturally level in a week or so, but keep checking them!

By doing this simple posture exercise, your body machinery will have more room to operate and your upper body will not compress the vital organs in your chest and abdomen. Become aware of the importance of good posture and your body mechanics – pages 39 to 44.

Healthy Walking is the King of Exercise

Walking is actually like a series of falls aborted by muscular force. When you realize this, you can better understand why it is so important to the health of your spine to walk correctly. When you *walk tall*, with a full-length lifted-up spine, the shock absorbers of your spinal column (*cartilage plates and disks*) have room to function well. Your spine will act as a spring, protecting the spinal cord and brain from the jolts of each step.

Continued pavement pounding takes its toll on spinal resiliency by subjecting your shock absorbers to undue stress. Shoes with low rubber heels and flexible rubber soles, help to cushion the shock. Your feet are springy levers that carry the weight of your body forward with each step. Although they need protection from hard pavement, they must not be confined or cramped; they need freedom of action in well-fitted shoes. (For discussion on how to fit shoes and take good care of your feet, see Bragg book *Build Healthy Strong Feet*. Dr. Scholl, a loyal Bragg follower who was active to almost 100 said *"The best foot program ever!"* See Bragg book pages 133-135.)

If you have pain or discomfort in walking, the three key points to check are your feet, shoes and spine. The Spine Motion Exercises and stretching exercises in this book will help greatly to make walking the buoyant, joyous exercise it is naturally supposed to be. You should gracefully swing along as though your legs began in middle of your torso, using the back, side and abdominal muscles as well as thigh, leg and foot muscles. Let arms swing rhythmically from shoulders. Hold head tall, and walk proud! Walking as Nature intended is the energizing *King* of Exercise that helps rejuvenate entire body!

How to Sit Properly

Slouching in a deep chair or sofa, just like slumping over a desk or table, distorts your spine. In different ways, this puts stress and strain in the wrong places (stretching some ligaments and muscles unduly, tensing others to compensate). This can jam some vertebraes together while pulling others out of place.

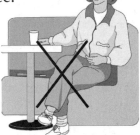

In sitting as well as standing, the same basic rules of posture apply from the hips upward, to the trunk and head, both supported by the spine and its interconnecting musculoskeletal structure. The base of your spine should be at the rear of the chair seat (which should be flat and straight), and your back against the chair back, which should fit the natural, gentle spine curves. The stomach then should

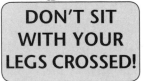

DON'T SIT WITH YOUR LEGS CROSSED!

be flat and firm (not relaxed outward), shoulders straight and head high. In other words, *stretch up spine and sit tall!*

Exercising, losing weight, and not crossing your legs when sitting can help keep varicose veins from getting worse. – www.nlm.nih.gov

The flat chair seat should be shorter than the thighs, so the edge of the chair does not press against the arteries under the knees. The height from seat to floor should be the length of the legs, with feet resting flat on the floor.

Don't cross your legs! Crossing one leg over the other throws the spine out of alignment and can bring on lower back pain and its problems. In a woman, this unhealthy habit can cause certain disturbances in female organs and, in a man, it may initiate prostate problems.

What if you're in a position where you can't choose your chair? Many medical professionals fault airplane seats, for example, for lacking proper lower-back support. Placing one or two small pillows behind your lower back *may leave you feeling a little less sore and stressed at end of flight*, says Dr. Helen Schilling, Health South-Houston Rehabilitation Institute in Texas. (*On planes we use ear plugs and eye cover.*)

Avoid Injury: Sit Correctly and Gently, Don't Flop, Slouch or Slump

43

Don't flop into a chair! Flopping into a chair, as most people do, brings extra shock to the vertebrae, wearing away cartilage plates and disks. Simply sitting down and rising from a chair correctly will exercise key muscles and ligaments and improve your posture. In sitting down, lower yourself into the chair lightly and gently, head forward and up, neck relaxed, spine lengthening and lower part of back widening, using your hip joints as hinges. Body weight is on the feet, ankles, legs and thighs – the powerful spring levers that gently lower your body into the chair. In rising, reverse the process, pushing upward from your feet, hinging from your hips, spine holding head and torso in alignment. Don't use your arms to push up from or lower yourself into a chair.

If you have been flopping, slouching and slumping, you may find these simple, correct methods difficult at first. Once you train yourself to sit correctly, however, you will find it much more relaxing, and actually restful, because the body will be in a natural position. *Start now!*

People who make positive improvements in their daily lifestyles habits significantly reduce the risk of back problems, cancer and heart disease.

Be a Bragg Crusader - copy and share with family, friends, clubs, etc.

WHERE DO YOU STAND?

POSTURE CHART

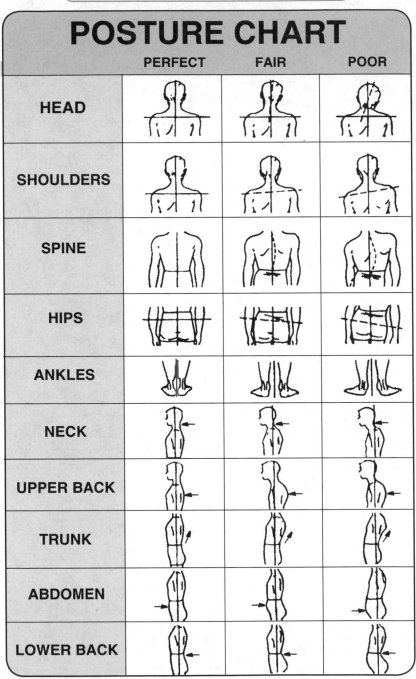

	PERFECT	FAIR	POOR
HEAD			
SHOULDERS			
SPINE			
HIPS			
ANKLES			
NECK			
UPPER BACK			
TRUNK			
ABDOMEN			
LOWER BACK			

44

Your posture carries you through life from your head to your feet.
This is your human vehicle and you are truly a miracle! Cherish, respect
and protect it by living The Bragg Healthy Lifestyle. – Patricia Bragg

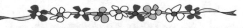

Remember – Your posture can make or break your health!

Keep Your Spine Aligned in Bed

Speaking of restful relaxation, your spine must be in proper alignment while you are lying down, whether for a rest, nap or good night's sleep. After all, we spend about a third of our lives sleeping! Sleeping on the wrong kind of mattress can throw your spine out of alignment.

A *soft, sagging mattress* fails to give proper support to the heaviest part of the body, the pelvic region and thus causes the spine to curve toward the side on which the person is sleeping. A completely rigid mattress causes curvature in the opposite direction because it does not give sufficiently to accommodate the wider hip and shoulder areas. Neither gives the back or spine the proper kind of support when lying on the back or stomach. Before buying a mattress, lie on it – see how you like it. You do not need box springs; just put mattress on a wood platform. A memory foam mattress topper can also greatly increase comfort, I just got one. It is great!

CHECK YOUR MATTRESS

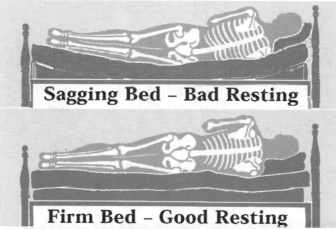

Sagging Bed – Bad Resting

Firm Bed – Good Resting

While sleeping, you recharge your battery you ran down during the day. The right kind of mattress is important. It's better to sleep on the mattress, than in it.

HEALTHY NERVE POWER: For extra "nerve power" insurance, take daily high-stress B complex, and a multi vitamin-mineral with calcium and magnesium. Also, to relax and sleep better, try melatonin, magnesium, calcium & Sleepytime herbal tea – natural relaxers that you can take before bedtime instead of sleeping pills.

Look for a semi-rigid mattress, firm and flat (one with sufficient resilience to allow shoulder and pelvic bones to form their own natural hollows), this helps keep spinal column in natural alignment. Placing wide bed board between mattress and springs converts most mattresses (except innerspring mattress) into a semi-rigid type your spine needs.

Noting that one doctor called the innerspring mattress *the devil's own work and a misbegotten gift of civilization.* The well-known orthopedist Dr. Philip Lewin, in his book *The Back and Its Disorders,* recommends a felted cotton, hair or sponge rubber mattress. He also advises to *stand tall, sit tall* and adds, *lie tall and on back is best to align spine.* If on back, roll small towel to support lower back and pillow under knees. Sleep with slanted, cradle pillow that elevates head (*it's healthier*). If on side, put pillow between knees. Before sleep relax all muscles, go limp, let yourself feel heavy on bed. Never let one part of body press on the other as this impedes circulation, keep arms and legs apart. Neck tension is often due to tensed facial muscles, so think pleasant thoughts that make you feel like smiling.

If you have difficulty getting sound, relaxed sleep, see some suggestions on page 70 and in *The Bragg Healthy Lifestyle* and *Nerve Force* book. See booklist pages 133-135.

Think Before Lifting to Protect Back Health!

Physicians confirm that spine stretching is imperative for everything from prevention of injury to flexibility and *strength. Murray C. Oransky, M.S., P.T., writes, The back muscles should be stretched daily, along with all muscle groups around both hips, as these muscles connect to the back and he stresses the important relationship for us between our daily lifestyle habits and our back pain.*

You may be using your back muscles improperly, or making these common mistakes: 1) standing in one position for prolonged period of time without elevating one leg (resting one foot on phone book or low stool), 2) bending over to pick something up without bending at hips and knees, 3) bending over to pick something up and twisting back while bending, or 4) carrying objects awkwardly too far away from the body.

Chapter 5

Stretching the Spine Promotes a Healthy Back and Body

Stretch to Avoid the Stretcher

As we noted earlier, you are *taller* when you arise in the morning, because a relaxing night's sleep allows your spinal column to stretch. Why doesn't it stay this way through the day? Why the need for special exercises?

Ordinary activities of the average person, from student to executive, housewife to movie star, simply do not use the spine to its full amazing capacity. Nature constructed the human spine to withstand an enormous amount of activity, constant use and even abuse. It is this very endurance that renders the ordinary activities, and even strenuous ones, inadequate for stretching the spine. Years of walking, riding, sitting, bending, turning, lifting and carrying have all made your spinal column so accustomed to bodily exertion that it is scarcely extended beyond the extremities of normal movement.

To a degree, Nature does replace the cartilage lost by constant wearing down, but there is rarely sufficient stretch of the spinal column in daily activities to separate the vertebrae the required amount. A little ground is lost each day, as in the case of Nature's restoration of tissue, blood, bone or anything else; this is, essentially, what is known as the process of ageing or *growing old*.

Nothing, of course, can bring the process of ageing to a 100% full stop. Unfortunately, most humans accelerate it by working against Nature, failing to obey Her laws. As we have discussed, the spinal column is a key factor in practically all of our life processes. That is why Spine Motion Exercises will not only stretch your spine, but also stretch your life in years and in the living of those years to the full enjoyment of vigorous health and vitality.

It's a lean, exercised, fit horse for the long, successful race of life!
Paul C. Bragg, N.D., Ph.D., Pioneer Life Extension Specialist

Natural Spine Motion

Animals practice natural Spine Motion. For Example: watch a dog or cat arching their back that spreads the vertebrae. A cat will lower the forepart of its body (*page* 61), extending its forepaws far forward and often they will twist their head and shoulders. This natural Spine Motion is the chief reason why these animals have such unabated energy over so long a portion of their lives. A dog whose normal life is eleven years, for example, will not show any noticeable ageing signs until its eighth or ninth year, and some will stay youthful until they are called to heaven. We have a healthy (*Eve*) 20 year old and (*Angel*) 18 year old.

We all have seen examples of people who begin to show early ageing in their 30s and 40s, but human beings were designed to stay active and energetic far longer than people might think. The human structure is mechanically adapted for full energies and activities at 70, 80 and 90 which is clear when we see people who are hale, hearty and fit, a spring in their step, clear of eye and keen of mind though well past three-quarters of a century.

Let us determine the proper leverages on the spinal column, apply them daily or every other day and watch premature ageing disappear. Spine Motion is so simple in application that one wonders why such a basic principle of youthfulness was so long in the discovery.

To repeat, there is nothing in physiology that responds in such a quick and positive manner as the spinal column does, when gently but sufficiently extended to its full elastic capacity. The muscles cannot alone cause a movement; their formation and fixed position limit the motion as well. That is why long study has been required to devise just the movements that will bring the spine into sufficient elongation in two different planes or directions, so the effect will be similar to the flexing given a string of beads that is turned and twisted in the hands.

Keep Healthy and Youthful Biologically
with Spine Motion Exercises and Good Nutrition.

The natural healing force within us is the greatest force in getting well.
– Hippocrates, Father of Medicine, 400 BC

48

Spine Motion Exercises Benefit Entire Body

These spine motions have been studied to successful conclusion and achievement. They have been tested exhaustively by the careful experimentation on, and observation of hundreds of people.

Now, thousands of men and women have benefitted by the marvelous stimulus of these Spine Motion and Posture Exercises. You may see and feel the results of spinal elongation and torque in a few weeks, often even in a few days. Family and friends will notice the big difference almost as soon as you feel the effects yourself.

Remember how, as a boy or girl, it was only parental rules for rest, afternoon naps or bedtime that could cause you to cease activities and relax? That was because your nerves were fully insulated, protected and independent. There was a full supply of cartilage to prevent wear and tear of your longest day from impinging on any set of nerves. The young spine had not begun to *settle*.

You can restore that condition to almost 100% at any age, permitting active use of the trunk muscles by these simple scientific exercises that impose no hardship.

Nerves are marvelously classified and grouped. We have learned how to concentrate in the building-up process in such fashion that vital organs can be helped separately and individually through Spine Motion, by exercising that particular portion of the spine from which the nerves that control these organs emanate.

Numbers of people, for example, have reported how these Spine Motions, especially #5 (on page 54), have given them magical relief from sluggish bowels, securing perfect regularity. This is due not only to relief from pressure on the nerves, but also to the fact that the motion of the pelvis aids elimination by making the large intestine twist and coil about and squeeze at the sharper turns where waste is so apt to accumulate.

Many such bonuses come from these Spine Motion Exercises. By scientifically stretching your spine, you will at the same time strengthen the muscles and ligaments supporting it, thus helping to hold the elongation and greatly improving your posture. Circulation and nerve energy will be stimulated throughout your body. Digestion will improve, as pressure on controlling nerves is relieved, and as organs become more firmly supported in correct position. You will breathe deeper, giving your body cells more of that priceless *invisible food*, oxygen.

Make Every Spine Motion Exercise Count

It is essential to put form into the performance of these exercises. The entire set of motions will not consume a consequential amount of time, nor will they cause more than momentary fatigue, so don't slide through them. Just as the routine movements of daily living are inadequate in keeping the spine limber and long, so would be a perfunctory performance of even these special movements.

You must throw a full measure of energy and enthusiasm into these Spine Motion Exercises, but don't overdo! For the first week or so, do the exercises slowly: feel your way, stopping short of the point of pain or fatigue. You will find this point extending day by day, as nervous energy is released and muscles strengthen.

When you first start limbering up the back, you may have some muscle soreness, but don't stop exercising. After a few days of continuous daily periods of exercise, the muscle soreness will disappear. Soon, you will find great satisfaction in doing these spinal exercises and the beneficial effects will amaze you. Now, let's get started! There are five main Bragg Spine Motion Exercises, each different in effect although similar in general aspects. Take a momentary rest between each one, but do the entire series.

Management and prevention of back pain begin by understanding the neutral spine position. Three natural curves are present in a healthy spine. The neck, or cervical spine, curves slightly inward. The mid back, or the thoracic spine, is curved outward. The low back, or the lumbar spine, curves inward again. The neutral alignment is important in helping to cushion the spine from too much stress and strain. Learning how to maintain a neutral spine position also helps you move safely during activities like sitting, walking and lifting.
– Medical Multimedia Group, at www.sechrest.com

Here Are Five Bragg Spine Motion Exercises:

Now, let's get you started with these five main Spine Motion Exercises. Each one is different in effect, though they all effectively stretch your spine for better health. Take a momentary rest between each one, but do the entire series.

Spine Motion Exercise #1

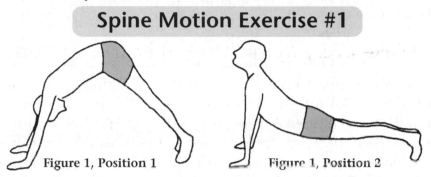

Figure 1, Position 1   Figure 1, Position 2

This first Spine Motion applies specifically to nerves that affect head and eye muscles. A reflex of the same motion affects a set of nerves that go to the stomach and bowels. Thus, in one movement, we attack eye strain, headache, indigestion and poor assimilation.

Lie face down on the floor. Now, rise to an arched position in which you rest on hands and toes with the back highly arched (see Figure 1, Position 1). The pelvis will be higher than the head. Feet are spread about 15 inches apart. Knees and elbows must be kept stiff.

Now, drop the pelvis almost to the floor (See Figure 1, Position 2). Remember: keep elbows and knees stiff (this is essential to impart the proper spinal stretch). As you lower the back, gently bring your head back; raise it as you lower the body. This is not a fast motion; take time in its execution. Dip to the extreme low, rise high again, arching the back all you can; down again . . . up, and down. If you do this motion correctly, you will find that a few times are enough. If only you could see what is going on along the spinal column during this jackknife action, you would know the relaxation and great relief imparted to the nerves all along the line.

51

Cats are graceful, coordinated and instinctively stretch to keep muscles tuned and joints flexible. Notice how cats feel the stretch, test the tension, relax and focus on the stretch. Order famous book, Stretching, by Bob Anderson, World's top Stretching Coach and Bragg follower. His wife did these sketches. Bob also gives Bragg Breathing Exercises at his sports seminars. www.stretching.com

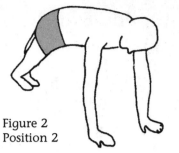

Figure 2
Position 2

Spine Motion Exercise #2

This second Spine Motion is designed to stimulate the nerves leading to the liver and kidneys. It can bring relief from many of the nervous conditions that are manifested in subnormal functioning of these vital organs. A sluggish liver and nonelastic kidneys, prematurely aged, for which there is no real excuse, will respond with surprising swiftness to spinal torque or twist. This exercise helps bring these organs quickly to a healthier state of vigorous function.

This motion starts in the same arched position as #1 (Figure 1, Position 1): face down, weight resting on hands and toes, back highly arched, with elbows and knees stiff.

Now, swing the pelvis slowly from one side to the other, to the very limit of your ability in each move to the right, then to the left, back and forth (Figure 2, Position 2). This motion should be done slowly. Always think of the s-t-r-e-t-c-h we must give the spinal column.

At first, you will find this motion tiring. It will grow steadily easier to do, not so much because of muscular development as because of vastly improved nerve organization. It should never become perfectly easy. This is more than a simple swaying of your body; you must make every one of the long row of vertebrae pull away from those adjoining them.

Researchers have discovered that the more healthy habits an individual practices, the longer they live and the healthier they are!
– Elizabeth Vierck, Health Smart

People who follow healthy living habits in early adulthood spend less time coping with disability in the years before their death. – Stanford University

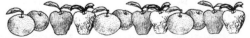

Nature's Wonder Working Phytonutrients Help Prevent Cancer
Make sure to get your daily dose of these naturally occurring, cancer fighting biological substances, that are abundant in apples, cabbage, onions, garlic, beans, legumes, soybeans, cauliflower, broccoli, citrus fruits, etc. The winner is the tomato, which alone contains about 10,000 different phytochemicals!

52

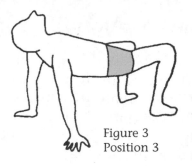

Figure 3
Position 3

Spine Motion Exercise #3

In this third Spine Motion, the entire spinal column is flexed from top to base. Every nerve center is stimulated. The pelvic region is specifically helped. This motion also strengthens those muscles attached to the spine that are most helpful in retaining the vertebrae in this improved and elongated position, that stimulates the growth of the intervertebral cartilage.

Take a new starting position for this motion. Sit down on the floor; then, raise the pelvis up by placing hands at sides (palms down) and drawing in feet about 12 inches. You are now resting your weight on the flats of your hands and feet, with pelvis and back up off the floor.

Raising the body, let the spine be horizontal as you finish the upward movement (see Figure 3, Position 3). Now, go down to the starting position, but lowering yourself to just above the floor. Go up once more, then down, etc. Two of the many remarkable benefits are the strengthening of the muscles and the spine.

53

Bragg Posture Exercise Gives Instant Youthfulness

Before a mirror, stand up, feet ten inches apart, stretch up spine. Tighten buttocks and suck in stomach muscles, lift up rib cage, put chest out, shoulders back, and chin up slightly. Line body up straight (nose plumbline straight to belly button), drop hands to sides and swing arms to normalize your posture. Do this posture exercise daily and miraculous changes will happen! You are retraining and strengthening your muscles to stand straight for health and youthfulness. Remember when you slump, you also cramp your precious machinery. This posture exercise will retrain your frame to sit, stand and walk tall for supreme health, fitness and longevity!

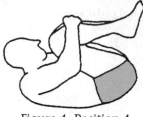

Figure 4, Position 4

Spine Motion Exercise #4

The fourth Spine Motion brings particular force to bear at the curve of the spine where nerves affecting the stomach are clustered. This motion also has the greatest efficiency of the whole series in the actual lengthening of the spine from top tip to end bottom tip. The results are felt in overall general improvement. After all, it is the general stretching of the entire spinal column that brings the whole system to balanced efficiency.

Lie on the floor on your back, hands at sides. Bend knees and bring to chest position, clasping arms around the legs a few inches below the knees. Now pull the knees and thighs tightly against the chest. At the same time, raise the head and try to touch the chin to the knees (Figure 4, Position 4). Hold this squeezing position for at least five seconds. Relax and then repeat.

54

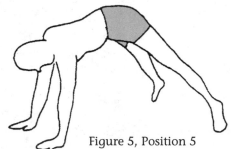

Figure 5, Position 5

Spine Motion Exercise #5 - A & B

In addition to its spine-stretching benefits, this fifth Spine Motion A & B brings speedy relief to sluggish bowels and organs both by nerve stimulation and exercise to the colon.

A Assume Position 1 by lying face down on floor, then rising to arched position, resting on hands and toes, the back highly arched up, pelvis higher than the head (Figure 5 Position 5). Now, walk all around on all-fours.

B The baby-crawl exercise on knees and hands also helps tone stomach muscles, etc. especially after childbirth. (Oil Billionaire H. L. Hunt, a Bragg follower, did this exercise daily and said it kept his spine and machinery healthier.)

Regular physical activity is part of a healthy lifestyle and spine. Apply variety, balance and moderation to your exercise program to normalize weight and for overall fitness. Exercises should build cardiovascular endurance, muscular strength, bone strength and flexibility of the entire body and especially the spine.

How Many Times and How Often?

The number of times you do each of these Spine Motion Exercises will rest with you individually. At first, three to five times for each Spine Motion will extend you amply. In a day or two, increase the count to five times or more. Since these motions are entirely new, you might experience some muscular stiffness during the first few days; this will pass. After it does, when spine and muscles and ligaments become more limber, a normally strong person will find ten times for each exercise no more difficult than were the three times of the first day.

How long to continue this series of Bragg Posture and Spine Motion Exercises? In the beginning, your spine-stretching routine should be a regular daily program. After you show marked improvement, two to three times weekly usually is sufficient to keep spine flexible.

Some people report that the very first session with Spine Motion Exercises has brought every apparent benefit promised, but it usually requires a week to see and start to feel the change. It is two to three weeks before the ground gained begins to take hold and assumes permanence of effect. Remember your spine is a miracle!

Please bear in mind that the settling down process of the spine has been a matter of years. It is not a condition you can overcome in a day. It takes time, and these Spine Motion Exercises give the spine time to stay stretched and stimulate cartilage growth and healing. Faithful daily practice of these exercises allows quick growth of cartilage under favorable conditions, thus securing the widened spaces between the vertebrae for a more healthy spine.

THE HEALTH LAWS OF LIFE

Man's body was created according to the laws of chemistry and physics, which are the Creator's own laws. They never vary. His law is written upon every nerve, muscle and every faculty that has been entrusted to us. These laws govern the cells, tissues and organs of the body as they carry on their various busy functions. They operate largely through the complex network of nerves that run throughout the body. They act through the central nervous system, from which nerve impulses originate, and through the autonomic nervous system, that part of the network not under the direct control of the will.
– Henry W. Vollmer, M.D.

The Body's Main Nourishing Arteries & Veins –
You Are A Walking, Talking, Human Miracle Machine

Arteries

Veins

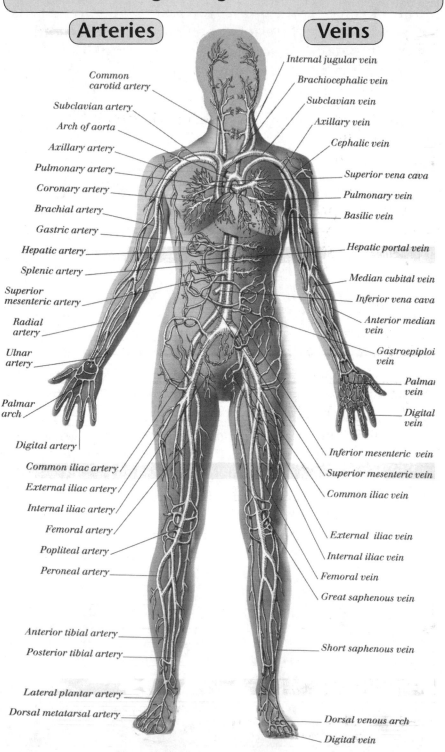

Common carotid artery

Subclavian artery

Arch of aorta

Axillary artery

Pulmonary artery

Coronary artery

Brachial artery

Gastric artery

Hepatic artery

Splenic artery

Superior mesenteric artery

Radial artery

Ulnar artery

Palmar arch

Digital artery

Common iliac artery

External iliac artery

Internal iliac artery

Femoral artery

Popliteal artery

Peroneal artery

Anterior tibial artery

Posterior tibial artery

Lateral plantar artery

Dorsal metatarsal artery

Internal jugular vein

Brachiocephalic vein

Subclavian vein

Axillary vein

Cephalic vein

Superior vena cava

Pulmonary vein

Basilic vein

Hepatic portal vein

Median cubital vein

Inferior vena cava

Anterior median vein

Gastroepiploi vein

Palmar vein

Digital vein

Inferior mesenteric vein

Superior mesenteric vein

Common iliac vein

External iliac vein

Internal iliac vein

Femoral vein

Great saphenous vein

Short saphenous vein

Dorsal venous arch

Digital vein

56

Chapter 6

12 Spine Motion Strengthening Exercises

In addition to the unique Bragg Spine Motion Exercises, here are some of the basic physical therapy exercises recommended by top orthopedists for strengthening the spine and its supporting muscles. We have selected a healthy dozen to include in this Spine-Fitness Program:

1 Neck Extension to Strengthen Upper Spine.

Stand in correct posture position, feet apart, muscles relaxed. Clasp hands behind head. Lean head forward, then attempt to push it backward as you resist with your hands. Do this for 6 seconds, counting one-thousand-one, one-thousand-two, etc. Repeat with head straight up, then with head as far back as gently possible. Gently stretch your neck as far as you can in each direction.

2 Back Stretching and Back Strengthening.

This exercise gives wonderful relief whenever your back feels tired. Stand up and stretch, feet slightly apart, rising on your toes and reaching upward with arms, then relax. Now bend over at the waist, knees slightly bent. Hold your legs with your hands behind the knees. Pull in your stomach muscles and attempt to straighten your back, while resisting back extension with your hands. Hold for 6 seconds, counting one-thousand-one, one-thousand-two, etc. Then relax, stretch and relax again.

3 Leg Extension for Strengthening Back.

Lean over a table, palms of hands flat on top near edge, elbows bent, standing far enough away so the head and torso bend comfortably parallel to table top, spine straight. Keep knees relaxed, feet flat on floor. Now, slowly raise one leg backward up high as possible. Hold for six seconds, counting one-thousand-one, etc. Slowly lower leg to starting position. Repeat with other leg. Continue, alternating legs, but stop when you begin to tire.

4   Neck Rolling to Strengthen Upper Spine

Stand in a comfortable correct posture position with no tension. Now, bring your chin to your chest, roll your head to one side (trying to make your ear touch your shoulder), continue roll toward your back (stretching the neck gently back far as possible), rolling on to other side (trying to touch that shoulder with that ear), then rolling head back to starting position. Do this exercise slowly, s-t-r-e-t-c-h-i-n-g the neck muscles, 20 times from right to left, then 20 times from left to right. This exercise is a must for desk workers, as it relieves muscular tension in neck and keeps the cervical vertebrae extended.

5   Rag Doll Exercise to Strengthen Entire Spine

Stand in comfortable correct posture position, feet about 18 inches apart. Pretend your arms are those of a rag doll, completely limp, letting them bounce limply as you swing your body from one side to the other, turning with each swing to look as far back as you can over each shoulder.

6   The "Old Favorite" Spine Bending Exercise

Stand erect with feet together. Raise hands over head, arms straight. Keeping the knees relaxed, bend forward and try to touch your toes with your fingertips. Gently stretch your torso downward to reach as far as possible, then return to the starting position. Next, with arms upraised, bend backward gently as far as possible, stretching the spine in the opposite direction. Return to starting position. Do this exercise at least 10 times.

7   Spinal Twisting Exercise

Stand in correct posture position, feet shoulder width apart. Extend arms to shoulder height at sides. Holding arms in position, twist your body from the hips as far as possible to the right, letting your eyes follow the back of the right hand, then as far as possible to the left. Try to see the same thing directly in back of you when twisting to each side. Alternating right to left, repeat 20 times.

He who can't find time for exercise will find time for illness. – Lord Derby

---

Our habits, good or bad, are something we can control. – Dr. E.J. Stieglitz

---

When you know what you want, and want it badly enough, you will find a way to get it!

8 | Endurance Test to Strengthen Lower Spine

Lie flat on your back on the floor, arms at sides. Keeping the knees stiff, lift your heels two inches off the floor and try to hold your legs and feet off the floor in this position for 60 seconds, counting one-thousand-one, etc. Each time you do this exercise, add a few more seconds. This really gives the lower spine a wonderful workout.

9 | Hip Rolling to Strengthen Lower Spine

Lie flat on your back on the floor, arms extended at sides at shoulder height, feet together. Raise the right leg vertically, toes pointed upward, knee straight, then swing and roll it to the left, touching toes to floor beyond fingertips of left hand. Return leg to vertical position, then lower it to floor. Repeat same exercise with left leg beyond fingertips of right hand. Do this exercise 20 times, alternating right and left legs.

10 | On-Side Exercise for Strengthening Spine

Lie on the floor on your right side, legs straight, arms comfortable. Keeping the knee stiff, raise your left leg straight up, then return it slowly to starting position. Now, bend the knee and bring your left thigh up against your chest and try to touch your chin to the knee. Do this ten times on the right side, then turn over to the left side and repeat ten times with the right leg.

11 | Arm-Hanging Spine-Stretcher

If you have access to a door or wall bar, do this exercise from a rung high enough for feet to clear floor. If not, use a door that is fully open and steady so it cannot swing, and place a towel over top edge so you can get a good grip. Now, grasp top of door (or rung of bar) and relax your body, letting it hang down free. If you use a door, bend your knees so your feet will be off the floor. Remember, this is an exercise for your back, not your arms, so make your body dead weight to s-t-r-e-t-c-h your spine. Hang like this for a few minutes, then relax briefly and repeat it at least three times.

I used to say, "I sure hope things will change." Then, I learned that the only way things are going to change for me is when I change! – Jim Rohn

---

A strong body makes a strong mind. – Thomas Jefferson, 3rd U.S. President

---

Prayer is the mortar that holds our house together. – Sister Teresa

12 Shoulder Rolls for Cervical Vertebrae

Stand in correct posture position, feet apart. Roll your shoulders up, then as far forward as possible, then down, then as far back as possible. Do this 12 times in a smooth, continuous circle motion. Pause briefly, then reverse the circular rotation for 12 times: up, back, down, forward. Increase daily from 12 to 30 times each way.

Take Exercise Breaks Throughout the Day

The first seven of these Bragg Spine-Strengthening Exercises can be done anywhere and anytime. All sedentary office workers should get up from time to time, stretch and do at least one of these exercises. You will return to your work refreshed with renewed energy. Instead of losing time, you will save it because you can work faster and better after an exercise *recharger.*

Dr. Henry L. Feffer, orthopedic professor at George Washington Medical School, stated: *The greatest strain on the intervertebral disks occurs while sitting, especially in an over-stuffed chair. The pressure per square inch on a disk is about twice as great when sitting as when standing, and this pressure is more likely to injure a disk if it doesn't have a good external muscular support, which is often the case in a sedentary person.* Dr. Feffer also stated: *Usually the chair that an office executive gives his secretary is much better for the back than the swivel chair he uses himself.* See web: www.gwumc.edu

If you are a sedentary worker, as millions of Americans are, use a chair that helps you maintain correct posture at all times. Be sure to get up out of that chair (correctly) at intervals to stretch your spinal column and strengthen your muscles. Get off the elevator several floors below your own and walk up final flights of stairs, head and chest up, spine in perfect alignment. Don't pull yourself up by the handrail; it's best to lean forward and up, pushing yourself from one stair to the next by the springy leverage of your hips, legs and feet.

If the next pasture looks greener, maybe it's getting better care!

Old age is not a time of life. It is a condition of the body.
It's not time that ages the body, it's abuse that does! – Herbert Shelton

60

Even if your work involves physical labor, remember that it is not necessarily the amount of exercise you do, it's the way you do it that counts. Remember the case of the *lumberjack* who *chopped* his spine out of alignment! If the muscles on one side of your spinal column are developed more than on the other, the spine can be pulled into a side curvature. Take time for exercises that *balance* those muscles required in your work.

If your daily activities are primarily those of running a household, home or office you will find your day easier and less fatiguing if you use some of these exercises during your day. Also, take *breathers* at intervals to stretch your spine and strengthen unused muscles.

Today many schools do not require regular Physical Education Classes. Teenagers and college students who have *outgrown* vigorous childhood games and recreation need to make a daily habit of practicing good posture and spine exercises. Spines can begin to *settle* even in your teens!

The Healthy "Cat Stretch" Exercise

Among the orthopedic exercises recommended by Dr. Arthur A. Michele, chairman of orthopedic surgery at New York Medical College and director of orthopedic surgery at eight other New York City hospitals, in his recent book *Orthotherapy*, is a healthy spine-stretcher that I think deserves your special attention. Although Dr. Michele calls it the *Long Body Stretch*, we call it the *Cat Stretch* because it reminds us of our cat's natural Spine Motion.

Kneel on the floor with your knees six to eight inches apart. Keeping your thighs perpendicular to the floor, bend forward from the waist, stretching your arms forward along the floor, let your forehead drop down as though to touch the floor, your torso sloping down from hips to elbows. Now, lower your chest as close to the floor as you can, pressing down for a fast count of ten. Return to starting (sloping) position for a count of five. Repeat as many times as you can in three to five minutes. This exercise stretches the entire spine and also limbers up the shoulder joints.

We have all seen animals, from cats to dogs to horses, lie on their backs and roll and wiggle their backbones with joy in soil or on the grass. According to another orthopedist, Dr. Lloyd Kingsbery, they are not merely scratching their backs; they are exercising their spines. He adapted this spine exercise for humans as follows:

Lie on your back, knees bent, feet about 18 inches apart, arms extended on floor at shoulder height, elbows bent with forearms parallel to head. Press the small of your back (lumbar vertebrae) flat against the floor, inching your hips downward, while your shoulders and head stretch back as your spine stretches out! Hold your body in this *natural traction* position as long as comfortable (count 1 to 20), relaxing when muscles begin to tire. Whether you feel tired or your back aches from physical or sedentary labor, these simple spine/back exercises help give you wonderful, refreshing spine-stretching relief.

Avoid Back Punishment – Protect Your Back

The single event that people think caused back injury may not be the problem. *Instead, it's almost a cumulative trauma*, warns Sheila Reid, rehabilitation coordinator at New England Spine Institute. *We go through years of misuse, and then there's one thing you lift, a fall or do that breaks the proverbial camel's back.* Even bowling, tennis, golf (one sided sports), etc. can also cause back problems.

A heavy shoulder bag can punish your back, too. *Putting extra weight on your shoulder unbalances you and, to compensate, many people twist their spines*, says rehabilitation specialist Dr. Karen Rucker of Virginia Commonwealth University. *It's best to take out things you really don't need.* This holds true also for shopping bags.

Long car rides can harm your back as well. The culprit is the phenomenon of whole body vibration. *It's a risk factor for lower-back pain*, says Dr. Malcolm Pope, director of the Iowa Spine Research Center. Simple steps you might take are: when the road gets rough, slow down (speed generally magnifies the effect of bumps), stop to stretch every hour of a long drive and, upon arrival, rest fatigued muscles a few minutes before unloading luggage.

Chapter 7

The "Gravity" of the Situation

Overweight Overloads Your Spine

When you consider that 1,300 pounds of pull are exerted on your spine and sacroiliac joints simply to maintain an erect posture, and that practically the entire weight of your vital organs is borne by the spine, you can understand why an excess burden of fat usually results in chronic backache. As we have discussed, your spine has enough jobs to do without having to carry a needless fat overload. I am sure you would rebel if you were forced to wear a sack filled with ten to a hundred pounds of rocks suspended from your waist at all times. Try it. That is exactly the kind of dangerous overload you force upon your poor spine when you are overweight.

Overweight exacts many other health penalties too! It over-burdens the heart with fatty tissue and forces the heart to strain with overwork in pumping blood through the additional miles of blood vessels. Often high blood pressure develops from obesity, also adult-onset diabetes. Fat deposits impede the functioning of vital organs, such as the kidneys and pancreas.

A belly hanging over the belt promotes back trouble and serious prolapsed stomach problems. The lower spine has to try to counterbalance that extra weight, says Dr. Schilling.

Back specialist Dr. Philip Lewin states the following in his research study on The Back and Its Disorders:

Overweight people are inclined to laugh off their excess pounds and dismiss it lightly. Doctors, however, regard it as a disease, and an insidious one at that. It is particularly treacherous because the fat person may falsely feel fit as a fiddle for a long time. But he can depend on it that his years will be decreased in direct ratio to the number of extra pounds of fat he carries. Insurance statistics prove it!

63

64% U.S. adults age 20-75 years are overweight, 30% are obese.

It's magnificent to live long if one keeps healthy, fit, alert, active and useful. – Harry Fosdick

Healthy Lifestyle Regimen for Reducing

The back is directly affected by overweight, and as a preventative, as well as a curative measure, anyone who has back troubles or who wishes to avoid them should watch those bathroom scales. After age 35, everyone is better off a few pounds underweight than overweight! See web: *walford.com*

If you are overweight as millions of Americans are, please don't delude yourself by believing in a *quick cure*. We have many people complain that they have tried this and that *crash or fad diet*, or one or another *sure way to reduce* without any lasting benefit. They have suffered various discomforts for short periods, losing some weight, often only to regain their lost weight and sometimes even more, as soon as the *crash diet* was over.

In our years as authors, nutritionists and physical conditioners, we have helped millions of men and women attain and maintain healthy, normal weight by natural methods. We know of no other sure way to accomplish lifelong weight control than by living a healthy lifestyle, establishing a regular regimen of diet and exercise that keeps your metabolism in proper balance. Metabolism is the intricate process by which your body converts food to energy. When you take in more fuel (food) than you burn up in energy (activities), the excess is stored as fat in the less used body areas.

A thorough explanation of how to lose weight and maintain it at a normal level is given in three Bragg Books, *The Bragg Healthy Lifestyle*, *The Miracle of Fasting,* and *Apple Cider Vinegar*. Many top Hollywood Stars and champion athletes, as well as millions of health students around the world, have successfully followed the Bragg Healthy Lifestyle teachings. If you are ten pounds or more overweight, or developing a tendency in this direction, these Bragg Books will be valuable additions to your health library.

It's strange that some men will drink and eat anything put before them, but they will check very carefully the oil put in their car.

Many people go throughout life committing partial suicide — destroying their health, youth, beauty, talents, energies and creative qualities. Indeed, to learn how to be good to oneself is often more difficult than to learn how to be good to others. – Paul C. Bragg

64

Healthy Diet and Normal Weight are Vital

According to the Centers for Disease Control and Prevention (CDC), women who weigh 20% more than they should are 30% more likely to develop osteoarthritis (the most common form of the disease) than their leaner friends. *More excess weight means more wear and tear on delicate body joints*, says Joseph Buckwalter, M.D., an arthritis researcher. There's scientific evidence that a plant-rich diet protects against arthritis on its own. The Arthritis Foundation reports that losing just 11 pounds could cut your risk of osteoarthritis in half!

Studies indicate you could also be at increased risk of osteoarthritis if one of your legs is longer than the other – a condition that affects one in five arthritis sufferers and can put excess pressure on the hip and knee of side with shorter leg. Experts say that chronic back or leg pain is one clue that your leg length may be off. Your doctor can measure it precisely, and a simple heel lift or chiropractic adjustment may be all you need to correct it.

One reason that being overweight is such a prevalent problem today, in every age group, is that most people eat too much of the wrong kind of food. In connection with overeating, Dr. Lewin makes this wise comment: *Two exercises, especially, are most beneficial to the reducer. The first is a shaking of the head from side to side when second helpings are passed, and the second is a pushing movement away from the table while still a little hungry!*

These maxims apply not only to the reducer, but to everyone wanting to maintain a normal, natural weight. We have never had an extra ounce of flesh on our bodies, and we have always made it a rule to get up from the table while still feeling a little bit hungry. As a result, we never feel sluggish and are always full of energy and vitality.

Despite the healthy tofu-and-avocado image Californians in 2009 enjoy across the U.S., over half the state's adults are still overweight. In 2002 researchers interviewed 4,149 people in all (1,772 men, 2,377 women) by telephone and found that 53% were overweight. Even back in 1990, 44.6% of Californians were overweight. Now in Nov. 2009, over 61% are overweight. – statehealthfacts.org

Maintain healthy, normal weight to avoid strain on your joints and back.

Another wise piece of advice from Dr. Lewin, which my dad also preached and practiced throughout his long, healthy lifetime, is: *A good reducing diet, one recommended by a health professional, gives the reducer all the necessary vitamins, minerals and nutrients necessary to maintain his body's health. If there is a chance that you are not getting enough essential food elements, it's wise to get some natural food supplements in capsule, powder, liquid or tablet form.* This is from an orthopedic speaking to patients whose backaches are due primarily to excess fat. Again, let me say it's sound advice for everyone to be fit and trim.

Maintain Healthy Natural Diet for Health

A diet of natural foods is the surest way to maintain normal weight and good health. In Mother Nature's design for living, she has provided perfectly balanced nutrition for every living thing in both the plant and animal kingdoms.

However, in attempting to redesign this pattern for their own convenience, humans have upset this balance, and are paying the penalty in loss of health. Modern civilization has concentrated masses of people in cities far from sources of natural food supply. The resulting need for mass transportation, storage and distribution of food has transformed the average diet into an artificial one, made up primarily of devitalized, processed, additive-ridden dead fast foods, which might satisfy hunger, but not the body's health demands. In the last 60 years, the American diet has deteriorated such that millions of children and adults walk around obese and malnourished, with low energy and weak, slumped spines. In a desperate effort to get a lift, millions resort to drugs; from slow killers (cola drinks, caffeine, alcohol and nicotine) to those that are more speedily fatal! Drug problems are growing deadly!

Is it possible to live on a natural diet in this polluted world? Yes, it is! It requires some dedicated, strong effort and wise discrimination, but the rewards are great. Isn't it worth your effort to exchange the misery of an unhealthy life for the joy of a vital, glowing, healthy life?

Stevia – World's Healthiest Herb Sweetener
Stevia drops (2 drops =1 tsp sugar) from South African herb plant, helps regulate blood sugar & lowers blood pressure, but doesn't affect normal blood pressure. Calorie-free, suitable for diabetics, safe for children & doesn't cause cavities. Helps mental alertness, combats fatigue & improves digestion. – stevia.com

Chapter 8

Choose Your Foods Wisely

Stop Eating Unhealthy Foods

When humans discovered that salt kept meat from spoiling, it became the first preservative and poison added to our natural foods. This happened so long ago that the majority of people have long thought of salt as simply a natural human food. It isn't! It's an inorganic, indigestible mineral – sodium chloride – not to be confused with organic sodium (in vegetables, fish, etc.) which the body assimilates and needs. Sodium chloride (common table salt) has no nutritive value, only harm. The body eliminates as much salt as possible, and stores any residue in water solution that bloats tissues, often with disastrous results. Today, the harmful effects of salt, still the most widely used food preservative, are aggravated by a host of new chemical additives and preservatives that are highly toxic and poisonous to the body, causing serious health problems.

67

The other major crime against natural foods has come about through refining or processing. Refined white flour has a long shelf life because it is actually dead; the vital raw wheat germ, one of Nature's richest sources of nutrition, having been refined out of it, leaves nothing but empty calories. The same sort of thing has happened to sugar, essential enzymes and vitamins having been eliminated by the refining process. The energy content of refined white sugar, as compared to raw honey, is like the burning of a sheet of newspaper compared to a steady wood fire. In a similar manner, processed meats and cheeses have been completely devitalized. Likewise, hydrogenated oils and margarines have been hardened into indigestible, insoluble lumps of dangerous clogging fats. So, for your health and life, take your glasses (if you need them) when food shopping and read all labels! Eliminate dead, embalmed foods from your diet! (See foods to avoid list on page 73.)

Self discipline is your golden key; without it, you can't be happy and healthy.
– Maxwell Maltz, M.D. author *Psycho-Cybrenetics* and a Bragg follower

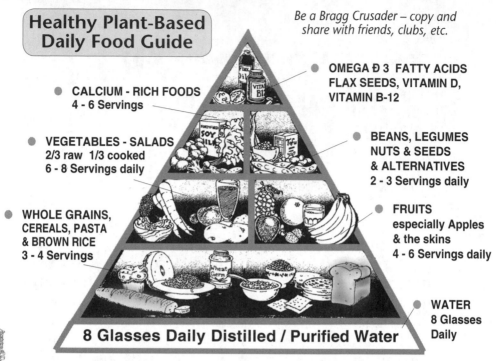

Healthy Plant-Based Daily Food Guide

- OMEGA Ð 3 FATTY ACIDS
  FLAX SEEDS, VITAMIN D,
  VITAMIN B-12

- CALCIUM - RICH FOODS
  4 - 6 Servings

- VEGETABLES - SALADS
  2/3 raw 1/3 cooked
  6 - 8 Servings daily

- BEANS, LEGUMES
  NUTS & SEEDS
  & ALTERNATIVES
  2 - 3 Servings daily

- WHOLE GRAINS,
  CEREALS, PASTA
  & BROWN RICE
  3 - 4 Servings

- FRUITS
  especially Apples
  & the skins
  4 - 6 Servings daily

- WATER
  8 Glasses
  Daily

8 Glasses Daily Distilled / Purified Water

The Healthy Plant-Based Daily Food Guide Pyramid is much different than other food guide pyramids you may have seen. This food pyramid is based on a more optimal diet eating plan of healthy vegetarian foods. There are no "junk foods" found in this pyramid. For those wanting to eat a healthful, balanced vegetarian diet, this pyramid provides excellent guide. It's in harmony with Bragg Healthy Lifestyle principles of optimal nutrition – see chart page 77.

At the foundation of the pyramid is distilled/purified water. We recommend distilled water as the optimal source of water to drink. It is the healthiest and purist type of water. We recommend drinking at least eight glasses of distilled water daily. Recognize that you also "eat your water" by eating healthy, organic plant foods as raw fruits and vegetables. The eight glasses you drink is in addition to the water you take in from your plant-based foods.

After the water base, the next pyramid level is whole grains. This includes all whole grain foods, including cereals, pasta, and brown rice. We recommend eating three to four servings a day of whole grains. An example of a serving of whole grains is one slice of whole grain bread, one-half cup cooked grains or cereal, or pasta. One ounce of a ready-to-eat whole grain cereal is also a serving in this group.

We next recommend eating at least six to eight servings of vegetables every day. Try to eat two-thirds of these vegetable servings raw and only one-third of your servings lightly cooked for optimal nutrition! Examples of a serving of vegetables are one-half cup of cooked vegetables, one cup of raw vegetables including salad, and three-fourths of a cup of vegetable juice.

We next recommend eating at least four to six servings of fruits daily. Here again we recommend to have most of your fruit servings raw, organic and uncooked. Examples of fruit serving include: one apple, banana, orange, grapes or pear; one-half cup of fruit, three-fourths of a cup of fruit juice, and one-fourth cup of sun-dried, unsulphured fruits.

It is important to have at least four to six servings each day of calcium-rich foods. You do not need to get your calcium from dairy products. There are plenty of other non-dairy, vegetarian calcium alternatives. (See chart page 94). These include soymilk, tofu and high calcium greens. Examples of serving sizes for the calcium-rich food group include: one-half cup of soymilk; one-quarter cup of tofu; one cup of raw or cooked calcium-rich greens like kale, collards, broccoli or Chinese greens; and one-quarter cup of almonds.

Beans, legumes, nuts and seeds, and vegetarian meat alternatives are excellent sources of vegetable protein in the vegetarian diet. It is recommended to have two to three servings from this group each day to meet your protein needs. Examples of vegetable protein servings include: one cup of cooked legumes (beans, lentils, dried peas); one-half cup of tofu; one serving of a vegetarian meat substitute such as a soy-based vegeburger or "veggie" meat slices; three tablespoons of nut butter; or one-quarter cup of raw nuts.

In order for you to get your essential fatty acids we recommend eating healthful fats from foods such as nuts and seeds (flax seeds and walnuts are excellent sources of omega-3 fatty acids), flaxseed oil, and Bragg Organic Extra Virgin Olive Oil. Taking dietary supplements that provide vitamin D and vitamin B12 are also recommended because sometimes these nutrients can be missing or at low levels in certain vegetarian diets if they are not properly balanced.

The Healthy Plant-Based Daily Food Guide provides you with nutritional guidelines that can be helpful in preparing healthful, delicious vegetarian meals for you and your family.

HEALTHY HEART HABITS FOR A LONG, VITAL LIFE

Remember, *organic live foods make live people. You are what you eat, drink, breathe, think, say and do.* So eat a low-fat, low-sugar, high-fiber diet of organic whole grains, fresh salads, sprouts, organic greens, vegetables, fruits, raw seeds, nuts, fresh juices and chemical-free, purified or distilled water.

Earn your food with daily exercise, for regular exercise, power walking, etc. improves your health, stamina, go-power, flexibility, endurance and helps open the cardiovascular system. Only 45 minutes a day truly can do miracles for your heart, arteries, mind, nerves, soul and body! You become revitalized with new zest for living to accomplish your life goals!

We are made of tubes. To help keep them open, clean and to maintain good elimination, add 1 tsp psyllium husk powder or oat bran daily – hour after dinner to juices, herbal teas, even Bragg Vinegar Drink. Another way to guard against clogged tubes daily is to add 1-2 tsps soy lecithin granules (*fat emulsifier-melts like butter*) over potatoes, veggies, soups and to juices, etc. Also take one cayenne capsule (40,000 HU) daily with a meal. Take 50 to 100 mgs regular-released niacin (B-3) with one meal daily to help cleanse and open the cardiovascular system, also improves memory. Skin flushing may occur, don't worry about this as it shows it's working! After cholesterol level reaches 180, then only take niacin twice weekly.

The heart needs healthy balanced nutrients, so take natural multi-vitamin-mineral food supplements, Omega-3 & extra heart helpers – mixed vitamin E, C, CoQ10, MSM, D-Ribose, selenium, zinc, beta carotene & amino acids, L-Carnitine, L-Taurine, L-Lysine & Proline. Folic acid, CoQ10, B6 & B12 helps keep homocysteine level low. Magnesium Orotate, Hawthorn Berry Extract brings relief for palpitations, arrhythmia, senile hearts & coronary disease. Take bromelain (from pineapple), multi-digestive enzyme & probiotics with meals – aids digestion, assimilation & elimination.

For sleep problems try 5-HTP Tryptophan (an amino acid), melatonin, calcium, magnesium, valerian in caps, extract or tea, Bragg vinegar drink & sleepytime herb tea. For arthritis or joint pain/stiffness, try aloe juice or gel, Braggzyme, Glucosamine - Chondroitin - MSM combo caps & shots, help heal & regenerate. Capsaicin & DMSO lotion helps heal & relieve pain.

Use amazing antioxidants – natural vitamin mixed E, C, Quercetin, grapeseed and grapefruit extract, CoQ10, selenium, SOD, Resveratrol, Alpha-Lipoic Acid, etc. They improve immune system and help flush out dangerous free radicals that cause havoc with cardiovascular pipes and health. Research shows antioxidants promote longevity, slows ageing, fights toxins and helps prevent disease, cancer, cataracts, jet lag and exhaustion.

70

Recommended Blood Chemistry Values

- **Diabetic Risk Tests:** • **Glucose:** 80-100 mg/dl • **HemoglobinA1c:** 7% or less
- **Homocysteine:** 6-8 μmol/L
- **CRP (C-reactive protein high sensitivity):**
    lower than 1 mg/L low risk, 1-3 mg/L average risk, over 3 mg/L high risk
- **Total Cholesterol:** Adults: 180 mg/dl is optimal; **Children:** 140 mg/dl or less
- **HDL Cholesterol:** Men: 50 mg/dl or more; **Women:** 65 mg/dl or more
- **HDL Cholesterol Ratio:** 3.2 or less • **Triglycerides:** 100 mg/dl or less
- **LDL Cholesterol:** 100 mg/dl or less is optimal
- **Blood Pressure:** 120/70 mmHg is considered optimal for adults

It's Important to Demand Healthy Foods

It is well worth the time and effort to read food labels – discard dead foods, and insist on fresh, live foods from reliable sources. We travel around the world for our Bragg Health Crusades, and we can always find enough fresh, natural foods to maintain our *Bragg Live Foods Lifestyle*. If you know what to look for, ask around and you can find it.

What the consumer strongly demands, long enough and loudly enough, the market supplies! Today (probably because so many people have health problems), there is a growing awareness on importance of healthy nutrition. Today an increasing amount of supermarkets have health sections, and also many have an organic produce section.

Our follower Texas oil billionaire H. I. Hunt made the LA Times front-page way back in 1972 showing his personal health food regime! A large photo showed the 83-year-old Hunt, reputed as one of the richest men in the world, crawling around on all fours (knees and hands) demonstrating the baby creeping Bragg exercise he did to strengthen his spine and back muscles after his back injury in an automobile accident (Hunt called us often).

Then, according to the Associated Press report, Hunt, who made a great part of his fortune from the processed and canned foods that bears his name and labels listing ingredients that included preservatives, demonstrated and expounded upon his personal health diet of fresh fruit and juices, nuts and fresh vegetables, grown in his own organic garden. He stated that these should be eaten raw and without salt, and that he avoids all white flour and white sugar, and eats only organic cracked-whole wheat homemade bread and raw honey. We hope it's not too much to ask that someday a giant food processor such as this will extend concern for his personal health to that of the consumers of his products.

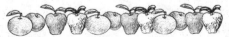

Healthy organic raw foods have wonderful abundance of potential life energy.

There is nothing which can hinder or circumvent a strong and determined soul that seeks with a passion health, usefulness, truth and success. – Ella Wheeler Wilcox

---

You're a Miracle – Self-Cleansing, Self-Repairing, Self-Healing – Please become aware of "YOU" and be thankful for all your blessings that take place daily!

The Law of Supply and Demand

The law of supply and demand is a natural one. It always works, sooner or later. The trend is visible already. As you and others join those who demand healthy, organic, "live" foods, the supply will inherently increase, as will the health of our country and civilization.

The same inventive technology, which created new problems of malnutrition in solving old problems of transportation and storage, has within itself the power to solve both the old and the new problems of nutrition in a healthful way. The development of refrigeration methods and increasingly rapid transport are now making it feasible for fresh foods to be brought to the marketplaces of the world in their healthy (organically grown) natural state, without having destroyed the natural vitamins, minerals and other vital nutrients.

This, of course, would mean that large food refining and processing plants would become obsolete, and therefore food manufacturers would undergo an interim loss while converting to new healthful methods that would benefit the consumer's health. This will not be done until the demand for healthful, natural foods becomes so great that major suppliers will have to fill it, or risk a permanent loss, instead of temporary loss.

New Non-Surgical Cure for Back Pain

Percutaneous Vertebroplasty – new nonsurgical, outpatient procedure for chronic back pain associated with spinal compression fractures usually caused by the osteoporosis progressive bone loss or from injury trauma to the spine. This procedure involves inserting a cement-like material into the center of collapsed spinal vertebra to stabilize and strengthen the bone. Under local anesthetic, a needle is inserted into fractured area of spine, using guided imagery (CT scanning and fluoroscopy) to fill the cavity with medical-grade epoxy. After the injection, the cement-like material hardens, creating a supportive structure that prevents further collapse and alleviates pain. This procedure takes under an hour and patients return home the same day. Of the 350 cases done in the past 2 years at Suburban Hospital in Bethesda, Maryland, by Dr. Wayne Olan, 85% of patients reported significant or total pain relief. This procedure also proved effective in treating fractures resulting from metastatic disease in younger patients.
See website: *www.mayoclinic.org/vertebroplasty*

Avoid These Processed, Refined, Harmful Foods

Once you realize the harm caused to your body by unhealthy refined, chemicalized, deficient foods, you'll want to eliminate these "killer" foods. Also avoid microwaved foods! Follow The Bragg Healthy Lifestyle to provide the basic, healthy nourishment to maintain your health.

- Refined sugar, artificial sweeteners (toxic aspartame) or their products such as jams, jellies, preserves, marmalades, yogurts, ice cream, sherbets, Jello, cake, candy, cookies, chewing gum, colas & diet drinks, pies, pastries, and all sugared fruit juices and fruits canned in sugar syrup. **(Health Stores have delicious healthy replacements, Stevia, etc, so seek and buy the best. Page 66)**

- White flour products such as white bread, wheat-white bread, enriched flours, rye bread that has white flour in it, dumplings, biscuits, buns, gravy, pasta, pancakes, waffles, soda crackers, pizza, ravioli, pies, pastries, cakes, cookies, prepared and commercial puddings and ready-mix bakery products. Most made with dangerous (oxy-cholesterol) powdered milk and powdered eggs. **(Health Stores have huge variety of 100% whole grain organic products, delicious breads, crackers, pastas, desserts, etc.)**

- Salted foods, such as corn chips, potato chips, pretzels, crackers and nuts.

- Refined white rices and pearled barley. • Fast fried foods. • Indian ghee.

- Refined, sugared (also, aspartame), dry processed cereals – cornflakes etc.

- Foods that contain olestra, palm and cottonseed oil. These additives are not fit for human consumption and should be totally avoided.

- Peanuts and peanut butter that contain hydrogenated, hardened oils and any peanut mold and all molds that can cause allergies.

- Margarine – combines heart-deadly trans-fatty acids and saturated fats.

- Saturated fats and hydrogenated oils – enemies that clog the arteries.

- Coffee, decaffeinated coffee, caffeinated black & caffeinated green tea. Also alcoholic beverages, caffeinated & sugared water-juices, cola & soft drinks.

- Fresh pork and products. • Fried, fatty greasy meats. • Irradiated GMO foods.

- Smoked meats, such as ham, bacon, sausage and smoked fish.

- Luncheon meats, hot dogs, salami, bologna, corned beef, pastrami and packaged meats containing dangerous sodium nitrate or nitrite.

- Dried fruits containing sulphur dioxide – a toxic preservative

- Don't eat chickens or turkeys that have been injected with hormones or fed with commercial poultry feed containing any drugs or toxins.

- Canned soups - read labels for sugar, salt, starch, flour and preservatives

- Foods containing benzoate of soda, salt, sugar, cream of tartar and any additives, drugs, preservatives; irradiated and genetically engineered foods.

- Day-old cooked vegetables, potatoes and pre-mixed, wilted lifeless salads.

- All commercial vinegars: pasteurized, filtered, distilled, white, malt and synthetic vinegars are the dead vinegars! *(We use only our Bragg Organic Raw, unfiltered Apple Cider Vinegar with the "mother" as used in olden times.)*

73

Allergies, Daily Journal & Dr. Coca's Pulse Test

Almost every known food may cause some allergic reaction at times. Thus, foods used in *elimination* diets may cause allergic reactions in some individuals. Some are listed among the *Most Common Food Allergies* (see below). Since reaction to these foods is generally low, they are widely used in making test diets. By keeping a food journal and tracking your pulse rate after meals you will soon know your problem foods. Allergic foods cause pulse to go up. (Take base pulse before meals and then 30 minutes after meals. If it increases 8 -10 beats per minute – check foods for allergies.) See web:*www.foodallergy.org*

If your body has a reaction after eating some particular food, especially if it happens each time you eat that food, you may have an allergy. Some allergic reactions are: wheezing, sneezing, stuffy nose, nasal drip or mucus, dark circles, eye watering or waterbags under eyes, headaches, feeling light-headed or dizzy, fast heartbeat, stomach or chest pains, diarrhea, extreme thirst, breaking out in a rash, swelling of extremities or stomach bloating, etc. (Read Dr. Arthur Coca's book, *The Pulse Test* – available: *amazon.com*)

If you know what you're allergic to, you are lucky; if you don't, you had better find out as fast as possible and eliminate all irritating foods from your diet. To re-evaluate your daily life and have a health guide to your future, start a daily journal ($8^1/2$ x 11 notebook pg. 115) of foods eaten, your pulse rate after meals and your reactions, moods, energy levels (ups and downs), weight, elimination and sleep patterns. You will discover the foods and situations causing problems. By charting your diet you will be amazed at the effects of eating certain foods. Dad kept a daily journal for over 70 years.

If you are hypersensitive to certain foods, you must omit them from your diet! There are hundreds of allergies and of course it's impossible here to take up each one. Many have allergies to milk, wheat, or some are allergic to all grains. Visit web: *foodallergy.org*. Your daily journal will help you discover and accurately pinpoint the foods and situations causing you problems. Start your journal today!

Most Common Food Allergies

- *MILK: Butter, Cheese, Cottage Cheese, Ice Cream, Milk, Yogurt, etc.*
- *CEREALS & GRAINS: Wheat, Corn, Buckwheat, Oats, Rye*
- *EGGS: Cakes, Custards, Dressings, Mayonnaise, Noodles*
- *FISH: Shellfish, Crabs, Lobster, Shrimp, Shad Roe*
- *MEATS: Bacon, Beef, Chicken, Pork, Sausage, Veal, Smoked Products*
- *FRUITS: Citrus Fruits, Melons, Strawberries*
- *NUTS: Peanuts, Pecans, Walnuts, chemically dried preserved nuts*
- *MISCELLANEOUS: Chocolate, Black Tea, Cocoa, Coffee, MSG, Palm and Cottonseed Oils, Salt, Spices and allergic reactions often caused by toxic pesticides on salad greens, vegetables, fruits, etc.*

Food and Product Summary

Today, many of our foods are highly processed or refined, robbing them of essential nutrients, vitamins, minerals and enzymes. Many also contain harmful, toxic and dangerous chemicals. The research findings and experience of top nutritionists, physicians and dentists have led to the discovery that devitalized foods are a major cause of poor health, illness, cancer and premature death. The enormous increase in the last 70 years of degenerative diseases such as heart disease, arthritis and dental decay substantiate this belief. Scientific research has shown that most of these afflictions can be prevented and that others, once established, can be arrested or even reversed through nutritional methods.

Enjoy Super Health with Natural Foods

1. **RAW FOODS**: Fresh fruits and raw vegetables; organically grown are always best. Enjoy nutritious variety garden salads with sprouts and raw nuts and seeds.
2. **VEGETABLE and ANIMAL PROTEINS**:
   a. Legumes, lentils, brown rice, soy beans, and all beans.
   b. Nuts and seeds, raw and unsalted.
   c. Animal protein (if you must) – hormone-free meats, liver, kidney, brain, heart, poultry, seafood. Please eat these proteins sparingly or it's best to enjoy the healthier vegetarian diet. You can bake, roast, wok or broil these proteins. Eat meat no more than 1 or 2 times a week.
   d. Dairy products – eggs (fertile, fresh), unprocessed hard cheese, goat's cheese and certified raw milk. We choose not to use dairy products. Try the healthier soy, nut (almond, etc.) and Rice Dream non-dairy milks.
3. **FRUITS and VEGETABLES**: Organically grown is always best – grown without the use of poisonous sprays and toxic chemical fertilizers whenever possible; urge your market to stock organic produce! Steam, bake, sauté or wok veggies for as short a time as possible to retain the best nutritional content and flavor. Also enjoy fresh juices.
4. **100% WHOLE GRAIN CEREALS, BREADS and FLOURS**: They contain important B-complex vitamins, vitamin E, minerals, fiber and the important unsaturated fatty acids.
5. **COLD or EXPELLER-PRESSED VEGETABLE OILS**: Bragg organic extra virgin olive oil (is best), soy, sunflower, flax and sesame oils are excellent sources of healthy, essential, unsaturated fatty acids. We use oils sparingly.

75

USA leads the world in heart disease, strokes, cancer and diabetes! Why? It's our fast trash high sugars, fats, processed foods diet.

The Bragg Healthy Lifestyle Promotes Super Health & Longevity

The Bragg Healthy Lifestyle consists of eating a diet of 60% to 70% fresh, live, organically grown foods; raw vegetables, salads, fresh fruits and juices; sprouts, raw seeds and nuts; all-natural 100% whole-grain breads, pastas, cereals and nutritious beans and legumes. These are the no cholesterol, no fat, no salt, "live foods" which combine to make up the body fuel that creates healthy, lively people that want to exercise and be fit. This healthy diet also creates energy, This is the reason people become revitalized and reborn into a fresh new life filled with joy, health, vitality, youthfulness and longevity! We have millions of healthy followers around the world proving that The Bragg Healthy Lifestyle works miracles for them! *Now it's your turn*!

Healthy Fiber for Super Health

- EAT BERRIES, surprisingly good sources of fiber.
- KEEP BEANS HANDY, probably the best fiber sources. Cook dried beans and freeze in portions. Use canned beans for faster meals.
- INSTEAD OF ICEBERG LETTUCE, choose deep green lettuces (romaine, bib, butter, etc.), spinach or cabbage for variety salads.
- LOOK FOR "100% WHOLE WHEAT" or whole grain breads. A dark color isn't proof; check labels, compare fibers, grains, etc.
- WHOLE GRAIN CEREALS. Hot, also cold granolas with sliced fruit.
- GO FOR BROWN RICE. It's better for you and so delicious.
- EAT THE SKINS of potatoes and other fruits and vegetables.
- LOOK FOR CRACKERS with at least 2 grams of fiber per ounce.
- SERVE HUMMUS, made from chickpeas, instead of sour-cream dips.
- USE WHOLE WHEAT FLOUR for baking breads, muffins, pastries, pancakes, waffles and for variety try other whole grain flours.
- DON'T UNDERESTIMATE CORN, including popcorn, corn tortillas.
- ADD OAT BRAN, WHEAT BRAN AND WHEATGERM to baked goods, cookies, etc.; whole grain cereals, casseroles, loafs, etc.
- SNACK ON SUN-DRIED FRUIT, such as apricots, dates, prunes, raisins, etc., which are concentrated sources of nutrients and fiber.
- INSTEAD OF DRINKING JUICE, eat the fruit: orange, grapefruit, etc.; and vegetables: tomato, carrot, etc. – *www.berkeleywellness.com*

Vegetable Protein % Chart

LEGUMES	%
Soybean Sprouts	54
Soybean Curd (tofu)	43
Soy flour	35
Soybeans	35
Broad Beans	32
Lentils	29
Split Peas	28
Kidney Beans	26
Navy Beans	26
Lima Beans	26
Garbanzo Beans	23

VEGETABLES	%
Spirulina (Plant Algae)	60
Spinach	49
New Zealand Spinach	47
Watercress	46
Kale	45
Broccoli	45
Brussels Sprouts	44
Turnip Greens	43
Collards	43
Cauliflower	40
Mustard Greens	39
Mushrooms	38
Chinese Cabbage	34
Parsley	34
Lettuce	34
Green Peas	30
Zucchini	28
Green Beans	26
Cucumbers	24
Dandelion Greens	24
Green Pepper	22
Artichokes	22
Cabbage	22
Celery	21
Eggplant	21
Tomatoes	18
Onions	16
Beets	15
Pumpkin	12
Potatoes	11
Yams	8
Sweet Potatoes	6

GRAINS	%
Wheat Germ	31
Rye	20
Wheat, hard red	17
Wild rice	16
Buckwheat	15
Oatmeal	15
Millet	12
Barley	11
Brown Rice	8

FRUITS	%
Lemons	16
Honeydew Melon	10
Cantaloupe	9
Strawberry	8
Orange	8
Blackberry	8
Cherry	8
Apricot	8
Grape	8
Watermelon	8
Tangerine	7
Papaya	6
Peach	6
Pear	5
Banana	5
Grapefruit	5
Pineapple	3
Apple	1

NUTS AND SEEDS	%
Pumpkin Seeds	21
Sunflower Seeds	17
Walnuts, black	13
Sesame Seeds	13
Almonds	12
Cashews	12
Filberts	8

Data obtained from *Nutritive Value of American Foods in Common Units*, USDA Agriculture Handbook No. 456.

Reprinted with author's permission, from *Diet for a New America* by John Robbins (Walpole, NH: Stillpoint Publishing)

1. Beet, celery, alfalfa sprouts
2. Cabbage, celery and apple
3. Cabbage, cucumber, celery, tomato, spinach and basil
4. Tomato, carrot and mint
5. Carrot, celery, watercress, garlic and wheatgrass
6. Grapefruit, orange and lemon
7. Beet, parsley, celery, carrot, mustard greens, garlic
8. Beet, celery, dulse and carrot
9. Cucumber, carrot and parsley
10. Watercress, cucumber, garlic
11. Asparagus, carrot, and mint
12. Carrot, celery, parsley, onion, cabbage and sweet basil
13. Carrot and coconut milk
14. Carrot, broccoli, lemon, cayenne
15. Carrot, cauliflower, rosemary
16. Apple, carrot, radish, ginger
17. Apple, pineapple and mint
18. Apple, papaya and grapes
19. Papaya, cranberries and apple
20. Leafy greens, broccoli, apple
21. Grape, cherry and apple
22. Watermelon (best alone)

Liquefied and Fresh Juiced Foods

The juicer, food processor and blender are great for preparing foods for gentle or bland diets and baby foods. Fibers of fresh fruits and vegetables juiced can be tolerated on most gentle diets. Any raw or cooked fruit or vegetable can be liquefied and added to non-dairy Rice Dream, nut or soy milks or broth or soups. Live, fresh juices super charge your body's health power! You may fortify your liquid meal with barley green, alfalfa, chlorella or spirulina powder for extra nutrition.

78

Bad Nutrition – #1 Cause of Sickness

"Diet-related diseases account for 68% of all deaths."

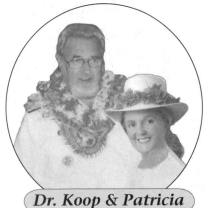

Dr. Koop & Patricia

Dr. C. Everett Koop, our friend and America's former Surgeon General said this in his famous 1988 landmark report on nutrition and health in America. People don't die of infectious conditions as such, but of malnutrition that allows the germs to get a foothold in sickly bodies. Also, bad nutrition is usually the main cause of noninfectious, fatal or degenerative conditions. When the body has its full vitamin and mineral quota, including precious potassium, it's almost impossible for germs to get a foothold in a healthy, powerful bloodstream and tissues!

Bragg Lentil & Brown Rice Casserole, Burgers or Soup
Jack LaLanne's Favorite Recipe

14 oz pkg lentils, uncooked
4 - 6 carrots, chop 1" rounds
3 celery stalks, chop, (optional)
2 onions, chop, (optional)
5-6 cups, distilled /purified water

$1^1/_2$ cups brown organic rice, uncooked
4 garlic cloves, chop, (optional)
$1/_2$ Tbsp Bragg Liquid Aminos
$1/_4$ tsp Bragg Sprinkle (24 Herbs & Spices)
2 tsps Bragg Organic Virgin Olive Oil

Wash & drain lentils & rice. Place grains in large stainless steel pot. Add water, bring to boil, reduce heat, then add vegetables & seasonings to grains and simmer for 30 minutes. If desired, last 5 minutes add fresh or canned (salt-free) tomatoes before serving. For delicious garnish add spray of Bragg Aminos, minced parsley & Bragg Nutritional Yeast Seasoning. Mash or blend for burgers. For soup, add more water. Serves 4 to 6.

Bragg Raw Organic Vegetable Health Salad

2 stalks celery, chop
1 bell pepper & seeds, dice
$1/_2$ cucumber, slice
2 carrots, grate
1 raw beet, grate
1 cup green cabbage, chop

$1/_2$ cup red cabbage, chop
$1/_2$ cup alfalfa or sunflower sprouts
2 spring onions & green tops, chop
1 turnip, grate
1 avocado (ripe)
3 tomatoes, medium size

For variety add organic raw zucchini, sugar peas, mushrooms, broccoli, cauliflower, (try black olives & pasta). Chop, slice or grate vegetables fine to medium for variety in size. Mix vegetables & serve on bed of lettuce, spinach, watercress or chopped cabbage. Dice avocado & tomato & serve on side as a dressing. Serve choice of fresh squeezed lemon, orange or dressing separately. Chill salad plates before serving. **It's best to always eat salad first before serving hot dishes.** Serves 3 to 5.

Bragg Health Salad Dressing

$1/_2$ cup Bragg Organic Apple Cider Vinegar
1-2 tsps organic raw honey

$1/_2$ tsp Bragg Liquid Aminos
1-2 cloves garlic, minced

$1/_3$ cup Bragg Organic Olive Oil, or blend with safflower, soy, sesame or flax oil
1 Tbsp fresh herbs, minced or pinch of Bragg Sprinkle (24 herbs & spices)

Blend ingredients in blender or jar. Refrigerate in covered jar.

FOR DELICIOUS HERBAL VINEGAR: In quart jar add $1/_3$ cup tightly packed, crushed fresh sweet basil, tarragon, dill, oregano, or any fresh herbs desired, combined or singly. (If dried herbs, use 1-2 tsps. herbs.) Now cover to top with Bragg Organic Apple Cider Vinegar and store two weeks in warm place, and then strain and refrigerate.

Honey – Celery Seed Vinaigrette

$1/_4$ tsp dry mustard
$1/_4$ tsp Bragg Liquid Aminos
$1/_4$ tsp paprika or to taste
2-3 Tbsps raw honey or to taste

1 cup Bragg Organic Apple Cider Vinegar
$1/_2$ cup Bragg Organic Extra Virgin Olive Oil
$1/_2$ small onion, minced
$1/_3$ tsp celery seed (or vary amount to taste)

Blend ingredients in blender or jar. Refrigerate in covered jar.

HEALTHY BEVERAGES
Fresh Juices, Herb Teas & Energy Drinks

These freshly squeezed organic vegetable and fruit juices are important to The Bragg Healthy Lifestyle. It's not wise to drink beverages with your main meals, as it dilutes the digestive juices. But it's great during the day to have a glass of freshly squeezed orange, grapefruit, vegetable juice, Bragg Vinegar ACV Drink, herb tea or try hot cup Bragg Liquid Aminos Broth ($\frac{1}{2}$ to 1 tsp. Bragg Liquid Aminos in cup of hot distilled water) – these are all ideal pick-me-up beverages.

Bragg Apple Cider Vinegar Cocktail – Mix 1 to 2 tsps Bragg Organic ACV and (*optional*) to taste raw honey or pure maple syrup (*if diabetic, to sweeten use 2 Stevia herb drops or pinch of Stevia powder*) in 8 oz. of distilled or purified water. Take glass upon arising, hour before lunch and dinner.

Delicious Hot or Cold Cider Drink – Add 2 to 3 cinnamon sticks and 4 cloves to water and boil. Steep 20 minutes or more. Before serving add Bragg Vinegar and sweetener to taste (*Re-use cinnamon sticks & cloves*).

Bragg Favorite Juice Cocktail – This drink consists of all raw vegetables (remember organic is best) which we prepare in our juicer: carrots, celery, beets, cabbage, tomatoes, and parsley, etc. (see more variety on page 78.) The great purifier, garlic we enjoy, but it's optional.

Bragg Favorite Healthy Energy Smoothie – After morning stretch and exercises we often enjoy this drink instead of fruit. It's delicious and powerfully nutritious as a meal anytime: lunch, dinner or take in thermos to work, school, sports, gym, hiking, and to park or freeze for popsicles.

80

Bragg Healthy Energy Smoothie

Prepare following in blender, add frozen juice cube if desired colder; Choice of: freshly squeezed orange or grapefruit juice; carrot and greens juice; unsweetened pineapple juice; or $1\frac{1}{2}$ - 2 cups purified or distilled water with some of following:

2 tsps spirulina or green powder, barley, etc.	1 to 2 bananas, ripe
1 Tbsp flax seeds (grind) (optional)	1 tsp soy protein powder
2 tsps blueberries, fresh or frozen	1 tsp almond or peanut butter
$\frac{1}{2}$ tsp lecithin granules	1 tsp raw honey (optional)
$\frac{1}{2}$ tsp rice bran	$\frac{1}{2}$ tsp vit C or emer'gen-C powder
$\frac{1}{2}$ tsp psyllium husk powder (optional)	$\frac{1}{3}$ tsp Bragg Nutritional Yeast Flakes
2 dates or prunes, pitted (optional)	$\frac{1}{3}$ cup soy yogurt or soy tofu

Optional: 4 apricots (sundried, unsulphured) soak in jar overnight in purified water or unsweetened pineapple juice. We soak enough for several days, keep refrigerated, also delicious dessert top with soy yogurt. Add seasonal organic fresh fruit: peaches, strawberries, berries, apricots, etc. instead of banana. In winter, add apples, kiwi, oranges, tangelos, persimmons or pears, and if fresh is unavailable, try sugar-free, frozen organic fruits. Serves 1 to 2.

Patricia's Delicious Health Popcorn

Use freshly popped organic popcorn (use air popper). Try Bragg Organic Olive Oil or melted salt-free butter over popcorn and add several sprays of Bragg Liquid Aminos and Bragg Apple Cider Vinegar – Yes, it's delicious! Now sprinkle with Bragg Nutritional Yeast Seasoning and Bragg Sprinkle (24 herbs & spices). For variety try pinch of cayenne pepper, Bragg Sea Kelp or fresh crushed garlic to oil mixture. Delicious served instead of breads!

Body Signs of Potassium Deficiency

🍎 *Bone and muscle aches and pains, especially lower back.*

🍎 *The body feels heavy, tired and takes effort to move.*

HAVE AN APPLE HEALTHY LIFE!

🍎 *Dizziness upon straightening up after leaning over.*

🍎 *Shooting pains when straightening up after leaning over.*

🍎 *Morning dull headaches upon arising and when stressed.*

🍎 *Dull, faded-looking hair that lacks sheen and luster.*

🍎 *The scalp is itchy and dry. Dandruff and some premature hair thinning or balding may occur.*

🍎 *The hair is unmanageable, mats and often looks straw–like, and is sometimes extremely dry and other times oily.*

🍎 *The eyes itch, feel sore and uncomfortable and appear bloodshot and watery. Also, eyelids may be granulated with white matter.*

🍎 *The eyes tire easily and will not focus as they should.*

🍎 *You tire physically and mentally with the slightest effort.*

🍎 *Loss of mental alertness and onset of confusion, making decisions difficult. The memory fails, making you forget familiar names and places you should easily remember.*

🍎 *You become easily irritable and impatient with family, friends and loved ones and even with your business and social acquaintances.*

🍎 *You feel nervous, depressed, in a mental fog, and have difficulty getting things done due to mental and muscle fatigue. Even the slightest effort can leave you exhausted, upset and trembling.*

🍎 *At times, your hands and feet get chilled, even in warm weather.*

81

Potassium deficiency is a proven contributing cause of many illnesses, including: Arthritis, kidney stones, atrial fibrillation, adrenal insufficiency, celiac disease, high blood pressure, coronary artery disease, ulcerative colitis, hypothyroidism, irritable bowel syndrome, Alzheimer's disease, multiple sclerosis, myasthenia gravis, Crohn's disease, lupus, atherosclerosis, diabetes and stroke. – Linda Page, N.D., Ph.D., *Healthy Healing* (visit website: www.healthyhealing.com)

THE MIRACLES OF APPLE CIDER VINEGAR FOR A STRONGER, LONGER, HEALTHIER LIFE

The old adage is true:
"An apple a day keeps the doctor away."

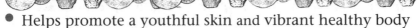

- Helps promote a youthful skin and vibrant healthy body
- Helps remove artery plaque and body toxins
- Helps fight germs, viruses, bacteria and mold naturally
- Helps retard old age onset in humans, pets and farm animals
- Helps regulate calcium metabolism
- Helps keep blood the right consistency
- Helps regulate women's menstruation, relieves PMS, and UTI
- Helps normalize urine pH, relieving frequent urge to urinate
- Helps digestion, assimilation and balances the pH
- Helps relieve sore throats, laryngitis and throat tickles and cleans out throat and gum toxins
- Helps protect against food poisoning & brings relief if you get it
- Helps detox the body so sinus, asthma and flu sufferers can breathe easier and more normally
- Helps banish acne, athlete's foot, soothes burns, sunburns
- Helps prevent itching scalp, baldness, dry hair and helps banish dandruff, rashes, and shingles
- Helps fight arthritis and helps remove crystals and toxins from joints, tissues, organs and entire body
- Helps control and normalize body weight

82

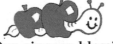

– Paul C. Bragg, Health Crusader,
Originator of Health Stores

Our sincere blessings to you, dear friends, who make our lives so worthwhile and fulfilled by reading our teachings on natural living as our Creator laid down for us to follow. He wants us to follow the simple path of natural living. This is what we teach in our books and health crusades worldwide. Our prayers reach out to you and your loved ones for the best in health and happiness. We must follow the laws He has laid down for us, so we can reap this precious health physically, mentally, emotionally and spiritually!

HAVE AN APPLE HEALTHY LIFE!

With Love,

Patricia

Braggs Organic Raw Apple Cider Vinegar with the "Mother" is the #1 food I recommend to maintain the body's vital acid-alkaline balance, plus digestion.
– Gabriel Cousens, M.D., Author, *Conscious Eating*

Ask Yourself These Vital Health Questions:

- How can I stop inorganic minerals and chemicals from hardening and turning my brain and body into painful stiffness and stone?

- How can I stop my body's joints and back from becoming painful, stiff and cemented?

- How can I help stop the formation of gallstones, kidney stones and bladder stones?

- How can I protect my arteries, veins and capillaries from the unnatural, hardening of arteriosclerosis?

- How can I prolong my youthfulness?

- How can I prevent sickness and premature ageing?

The answer is *drink pure distilled water!* For more details on why we say this, do read the Bragg book, *Water – The Shocking Truth That Can Save Your Life!*

The Miracle Life of Ageless Jack LaLanne

83

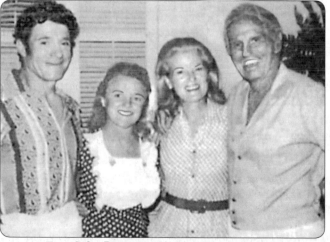

Jack LaLanne, Patricia Bragg, Elaine LaLanne & Paul C. Bragg

Jack says he would have been dead by 16 if he hadn't attended The Bragg Crusade. Jack says, *Bragg saved my life at age 15, when I attended the Bragg Health and Fitness Crusade in Oakland, California.* From that day, Jack has continued to live The Bragg Healthy Lifestyle, inspiring millions to health, fitness and a long and happy life! See his website: *www.jacklalanne.com*

Doubt destroys. Faith builds! – Robert Collier

The 70% Watery Human

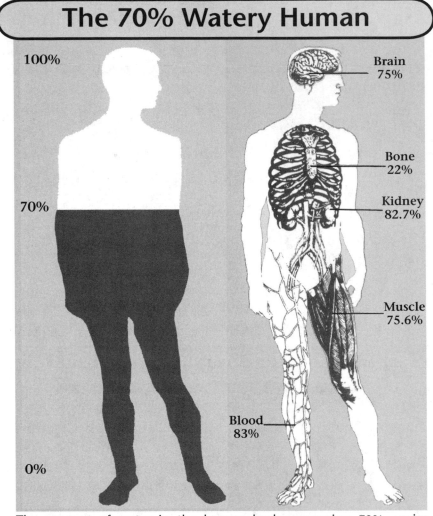

100%

70%

0%

Brain
75%

Bone
22%

Kidney
82.7%

Muscle
75.6%

Blood
83%

The amount of water in the human body, averaging 70%, varies considerably and even from one part of the body to another area (illustration on right). A lean man may hold 70% of his weight in body water, while a woman – because of her larger proportion of water-poor fatty tissues – may be only 52% water. The lowering of the water content in the blood is what triggers the hypothalamus, the brain's vital thirst center, to send out its familiar urgent demand for a drink of water! Please obey and drink ample amounts of purified water.

By the time you feel thirsty, you're already dehydrated. – American Running & Fitness Assoc.

Water Percentage in Various Body Parts:

Teeth	10%	Lungs	80%
Bones	22%	Brain	75%
Cartilage	55%	Bile	86%
Red blood corpuscles	68.7%	Plasma	90%
Liver	71.5%	Blood	83%
Muscle tissue	75%	Lymph	94%
Spleen	75.5%	Saliva	95.5%

This chart shows why 8-10 glasses of water daily is important.

84

Play it Safe – Drink Pure Distilled Water!

Pure distilled water is vitally important in following The Bragg Healthy Heart Lifestyle. Water is the key to all body functions including: digestion, assimilation, elimination and circulation, and to bones and joints, muscles, nerves, glands and senses. The right kind of water is one of your best natural protections against all kinds of diseases and infections. It's a vital factor in all the body fluids, tissues, cells, lymph, blood and all glandular secretions. Water holds all nutritive factors in solution, as well as toxins and body wastes, and acts as the main transportation medium throughout the body, for both nutrition and cleansing purposes.

Since your body is about 70% water, the blood and lymphatic system is over 90% water, it's essential for your health that you drink only pure water that's not saturated with contaminants, inorganic minerals and toxins. This water will transport vital nutrients to cells and waste from cells more efficiently. This allows the body to function correctly and stay healthier!

ORGANIC MINERALS Your minerals must come from an organic source, from something living or that has lived. Humans do not have the same chemistry as plants. Only the living plant has the ability to extract inorganic minerals from the earth and convert them to organic minerals for your body to absorb and utilize.

INORGANIC MINERALS Inorganic minerals and toxic chemicals in water can create these problems:

- Causes arthritis, bone spurs and painful calcified formations in the joints.

- Harden the liver.

- Cause kidney and gallstones.

- Clog and harden the veins, capillaries and arteries.

- Inorganic minerals and the toxic chemicals in water clog the arteries and small capillaries that are needed to feed and nourish your brain with oxygenated blood. The result is gradual loss of alertness, memory and danger of strokes and senility.

85

Cocktail of Toxic Chemicals

Chlorine, fluoride, calcium carbonate cadmium, aluminum, trihalomethanes, chloroform, arsenic copper, lead and unpleasant taste

Tap-Water Average Contents

Water is the Key to All Body Functions

- Heart
- Circulation
- Digestion
- Bones & Joints
- Muscles
- Metabolism
- Assimilation
- Elimination
- Nerves
- Glands
- Sex
- Energy

Pure Water is Important for Super Health

People who ingest a sufficient amount of the right kinds of liquids (distilled water, fresh fruits and vegetables and their juices) have better body functioning and circulation overall, which are most important to Super Health and Long Life.

You have 15 billion powerful brain cells and the brain is 80.5% water. We strongly believe the right kind of water in sufficient amounts helps improve your mind and brain power and makes you think better and more accurately!

We also think that the excessively nervous and/or mentally upset person is so obsessed with his own worries and *hang-ups* that he just forgets to drink sufficient pure water. Instead, he dopes himself with alcohol, tea, coffee, cola and sugar drinks which only complicate his nervous condition by introducing burning, toxic acid into his stomach with no food or water to dilute it. So on top of his nervousness and depression, he suffers from heartburn, sour acid stomach, gas, bloating, enervation and low energy. In place of sufficient pure water, he again dopes up on stimulants, coffee, soft drinks, cigarettes, aspirin, antacids, etc.

Remember that the whole body, heart, nerves and colon need the correct amount of water to function properly and smoothly. You can plainly see that it is possible to suffer from water starvation. Here's a simple way to help yourself to better health – daily drink 8 glasses of distilled water!

86

Shocking Mutations & Death from Polluted Water Must Stop!

Deadly chemical pollution is not only mutating but killing millions of wildlife, fish, etc. worldwide. One USA example: Children in Minnesota discovered and caught frogs displaying horrible mutations, including eyes growing on their knees, four hind legs, etc. Scientists have now determined that unidentified toxic chemicals in the pond and ground water caused these terrible mutations!

He who understands nature walks with God. – Edgar Cayce

"Good Earth" Founder Thanks Bragg Books

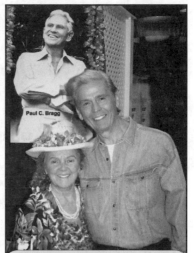

Bill Galt, the founder of The Good Earth Restaurant chain, charged himself with Super Health and changed his entire life after reading Bragg books *Miracle of Fasting* and *The Bragg's Vegetarian Recipes*. His entire family followed The Bragg Healthy Lifestyle. Their friends and associates wanted to know what was the cause of the miraculous changes they saw

Patricia with Bill Galt & Paul Bragg's Picture

in the Galts! Their friends wanted what they had – Super Health! Bill and his family started a tiny restaurant that served only lunches. An overnight success, they were soon serving a full menu all day. Soon they expanded their base of operations and opened a chain of health restaurants, all serving delicious food based on The Bragg Healthy Lifestyle! We were blessed to have a Good Earth Restaurant in Santa Barbara. Many Hollywood Stars often ate there, including the Jack LaLannes.

87

We Thank Thee

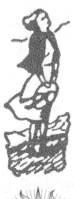

For flowers that bloom about our feet;
    For song of bird and hum of bee;
For all things fair we hear or see,
    Father in heaven we thank Thee!
For blue of stream and blue of sky;
    For pleasant shade of branches high;
For fragrant air and cooling breeze;
    For beauty of the blooming trees;
Father in heaven we thank Thee!
    For mother love and father care,
For brothers strong and sisters fair;
    For love at home and here each day;
For guidance lest we go astray,
    Father in heaven we thank Thee!
For this new morning with its light;
    For rest and shelter of the night;
For health and food, for love and friends;
    For every thing His goodness sends,
Father in heaven we thank Thee!
      – Ralph Waldo Emerson

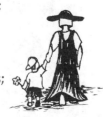

Take Time for 12 Things

1. Take time to **Work** –
   it is the price of success.
2. Take time to **Think** –
   it is the source of power.
3. Take time to **Play** –
   it is the secret of youth.
4. Take time to **Read** –
   it is the foundation of knowledge.
5. Take time to **Worship** –
   it is the highway of reverence and
   washes the dust of earth from our eyes.
6. Take time to **Help and Enjoy Friends** –
   it is the source of happiness.
7. Take time to **Love and Share** –
   it is the one sacrament of life.
8. Take time to **Dream** –
   it hitches the soul to the stars.
9. Take time to **Laugh** –
   it is the singing that helps life's loads.
10. Take time for **Beauty** –
    it is everywhere in nature.
11. Take time for **Health** –
    it is the true wealth and treasure of life.
12. Take time to **Plan** –
    it is the secret of being able to have time
    for the first 11 things.

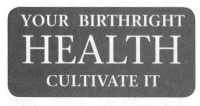

YOUR BIRTHRIGHT
HEALTH
CULTIVATE IT

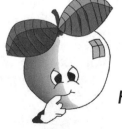

*Have an
Apple
Healthy Life!*

*Teach me Thy way O Lord, and
lead me in a simple healthy path. – Psalms 27:11*

Chapter 9

Eat Right to Build Healthy Bones

Osteoporosis Due to Faulty Diet

Remember that the bones comprising your spinal column and the rest of your skeletal system are living tissue and must receive the proper nourishment in order to be strong and healthy for your entire lifetime.

Basic bone structure, as we discussed previously, consists of a rigid outer sheath that gives the bone its shape and strength, filled with elastic, spongy material called marrow. Engineers have adapted this structural principle in the construction of buildings, finding that such supports as metal pipes that are filled with dirt, for example, are stronger, more enduring and resilient than solid, rigid structures. Usually these man-made structures, however, deteriorate with time. This is not so with the living bones of the human skeleton.

Our bones do not *grow brittle with age*. They become brittle, weak and porous because of deficiencies in diet. This condition is known as osteoporosis, from *osteo* for bone, *por* for pore and *osis* for disease, a *pore* being a small hole like those through which we perspire.

Although osteoporosis has long been considered an almost inevitable affliction of people over 50 years of age, the time element is not the basic factor. It is true that the longer you abuse your body by incorrect diet, inadequate exercise and insufficient rest, the greater price you will pay in the degenerative symptoms commonly known as ageing. However, this can happen at any stage of your calendar years. Look at the number of young men and women who are rejected from the armed services and from civilian work requiring good physical stamina, because of various physical deficiencies, from fallen arches to curvature of the spine (*due, in our opinion, primarily to the habitual American fast trash diet of the commercialized, dead foods, plus an unhealthy lifestyle*).

Natural Healthy Foods Prevent Osteoporosis

When we were doing nutritional research along the Adriatic coast of Italy, we found ageless men and women, advanced in calendar years but whose bodies were youthful, supple and bones firm, strong and resilient. Their diet consisted primarily of organically grown fresh salads, properly cooked vegetables, olive oil, dark breads, pasta and natural cheeses rich in calcium, vitamins and minerals, all essential for strong bones. In our extensive research on nutrition, we never found osteoporosis among active people who lived on a simple diet of live, natural healthy foods (see web: *www.calciuminfo.com*).

The American fast, trash diet, in addition to lacking vitamins and minerals, is also highly acid-producing, due to the high proportion of refined white sugar and white flour and animal proteins, which increase the acidity of the body with an adverse effect on the bones. Strong bones require an alkaline balance in the body metabolism, naturally maintained by a higher proportion of raw organic fruits and vegetables in the diet.

The worst villain is refined white sugar and its many products; there is no single food more devastating to the spine and other bones of the body. It leaches calcium, phosphorus, magnesium and manganese out of the bones, making them weak, porous and brittle. Candy, sweets and refined white sugar products and drinks are also prime causes of tooth decay. Since teeth are the body's hardest tissue, you can understand what refined white sugar does to other bones and cartilages (protective cushions between bones) of the skeletal system, including your spinal column (see web: *www.homocysteine.com*).

90

WANTED – For Robbing Health and Life

KILLER Saturated Fats	CHOKER Hydrogenated Fats
CLOGGER Salt	DEAD-EYED Devitalized Foods
DOPEY Caffeine	HARD Water (Inorganic Minerals)
PLUGGER Frying Pan	JERKY Turbulent Emotions
DEATH-DEALER Drugs	CRAZY Alcohol
GREASY Overweight	SMOKY Tobacco
HOGGY Overeating	LOAFER Laziness

Locations in the Body Where Osteoporosis, Arthritis, Pain and Misery Hit the Hardest

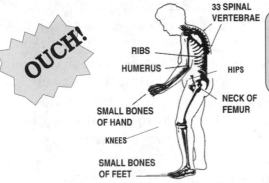

OUCH!

33 SPINAL
VERTEBRAE

RIBS

HUMERUS

HIPS

NECK OF
FEMUR

SMALL BONES
OF HAND

KNEES

SMALL BONES
OF FEET

OSTEOPOROSIS
**Affects over 30 Million
and Kills 400,000
Americans Annually**

Boron
Miracle Trace Mineral
For Healthy Bones

BORON – A trace mineral for healthier bones that also helps the body absorb more vital calcium, minerals and necessary hormones! Good sources are most vegetables, fresh and sun- dried fruits, prunes, raw nuts, soybeans and nutritional Brewer's yeast.

The U.S. Department of Agriculture's Human Nutrition Lab in Grand Forks, North Dakota, says boron is usually found in soil and in foods, but many Americans eat a diet low in boron. They conducted a 17 week study which showed a daily 3 to 6 mgs. boron supplement enabled participants to reduce loss (demineralization) of calcium, phosphorus and magnesium from their bodies. This loss is usually caused by eating processed fast foods and lots of meat, salt, sugar and fat and a dietary lack of fresh vegetables, fruits and whole grains. *(www.all-natural.com)*

After 8 weeks on boron, participants' calcium loss was cut 40%. It also helped double important hormone levels vital in maintaining calcium and healthy bones. Millions of women on estrogen replacement therapy for osteoporosis* may want to use boron as a healthier choice. Also consider the natural progesterone (2%) raw yam cream. For pain, joint support and healing use a glucosamine/chondriotin/MSM combo *(caps, liquid, roll-on or shots)*.

Scientific studies show women benefit from a healthy lifestyle that includes some gentle sunshine and ample exercise *(even weight lifting)* to maintain healthier bones, combined with a low-fat, high-fiber, carbohydrate, and fresh fruits, salads, greens and vegetable diet. This lifestyle helps protect against heart disease, high blood pressure, cancer and many other ailments. I'm happy to see science now agrees with my Dad who first stated these health truths in the 1930's.

91

*For more hormone and osteoporosis facts read pioneer John Lee, M.D.'s book – *What Your Doctor May Not Tell You About Menopause.* (amazon.com)

Your Spine Needs Organic Minerals

The only way to protect yourself against osteoporosis, or to restore weak, porous, brittle bones to a healthy state, is by proper nutrition. Given the proper tools to work with, the human body is self-healing and self-repairing, but don't expect overnight miracles. If you have been eating incorrectly for a period of time, it is going to take time to repair the damage after you make the change to a Program of Natural Nutrition. Start today! Eliminate the dead foods from your diet, and give your bones and the rest of your body the live foods on which they thrive.

For strong, healthy bones and a spinal column that really serves as the mainspring of your body, particular attention should be paid to the foods that supply the organic minerals essential to bone building. These are calcium, phosphorus, magnesium and manganese.

Calcium is important in reparation of all cells and the major component of the bones of the body. Ninety percent of the body's calcium is to be found in the skeletal system, where it is not only used as the main ingredient of bone structure, but also stored for use elsewhere in the body as needed. If your diet is deficient in natural, organic calcium, your bones will not only suffer from this lack, but they will become further weakened by the drain on their inadequate supply for other uses throughout the body. For example, during pregnancy the fetus draws on its mother's calcium supply, and if she is deficient, her teeth and bones suffer as well as the child's.

Although only 1% of the body's calcium is used by the soft tissues, it is vital to health, especially of the nerves. It is not just the spinal column that needs this organic material, but also the spinal cord itself. Usually, the most noticeable sign of calcium deficiency is extreme nervousness. Without enough calcium in the blood, nerves have trouble sending messages. Tension and strain result; it is impossible for the body to relax. This is apparent in children who are highly emotional. It shows first by an unpleasant disposition, fretful crying and temper tantrums, later to develop into muscular twitching, spasms and even convulsions.

Calcium Deficiencies Affect All Ages

Both adults and children (85% of Americans!) reveal calcium deficiencies by nervous habits such as biting their fingernails and restless body movements of hands, legs and feet (called restless legs syndrome), irritability and jumpiness. This calcium and magnesium deficiency can be a major contributing cause of adverse personality changes.

Fortunately, an adequate supply of calcium in the system has the opposite effect. In our years of experience as nutritionists, we have seen the meanest, most irritable, nervous people make personality changes for the better. We have seen miracle changes – happy, healthy, peaceful people, by following our Bragg Healthy Lifestyle of good nutrition and living habits. Also, calcium contains the natural material that causes the blood to clot. If we did not have calcium in our bloodstream, we could prick a finger with a needle and bleed to death!

Natural Calcium Sources (page 94) offers wide variety of this important mineral you can include in every meal. Protein foods high in calcium, for meat eaters, include organ meats like liver, kidneys, heart, etc.; natural, unprocessed yellow cheeses; fresh, fertile eggs. Stone-ground cornmeal, whole natural oatmeal and whole natural barley are fine sources; so are raw nuts and seeds. Green leafy vegetables abound in calcium: alfalfa sprouts, spinach, beet greens, mustard greens, collards, broccoli, kale, cabbage, cauliflower, dandelion greens, lettuce, also snow peas, carrots and cucumbers. Fruit sources include: oranges, sun-dried dates, figs, prunes and raisins.

Milk is Not the Best Source of Calcium

Most Americans believe milk is the best way to get calcium your body needs, but there are many reasons why this is not true (see web: *notmilk.com*). *First*: almost all American milk is both pasteurized (boiled) and homogenized to kill any bacteria that might make you sick. This process also reduces the available calcium in milk. *Second*: milk also contains an enzyme called lactose to which most people are allergic. The major symptom of lactose intolerance is mucus formation, but most people don't recognize this symptom as the allergic response that it is. Third: you must take into the account the herbicides, pesticides and fungicides that cattle ingest through their foods, and the hormones, growth stimulators, antibiotics and other drugs that are pumped into cattle to treat disease and maximize weight and milk production. All of these toxins are passed on to you through their milk. Avoid dairy products and fulfill your calcium requirements with some of these nutritious foods:

Calcium Content of Some Common Foods

Food Source	mgs	Food Source	mgs
Almonds, 1 oz	80	Kale (steamed), 1 cup	180
Artichokes (steamed), 1 cup	51	Kohlrabi (steamed), 1 cup	40
Beans (kidney, pinto, red), 1 cup	89	Mustard greens, 1 cup	138
Beans (great northern, navy), 1 cup	128	Oatmeal, 1 cup	120
Beans (white), 1 cup	161	Orange, 1 large	96
Blackstrap molasses, 1 Tbsp	137	Prunes, 4 whole	45
Bok choy (steamed), 1 cup	158	Raisins, 4 oz	45
Broccoli (steamed), 1 cup	178	Rhubarb (cooked), 1 cup	105
Brussel Sprouts (steamed), 1 cup	56	Rutabaga (steamed), 1 cup	72
Buckwheat pancake, 1	99	Sesame seeds (unhulled), 1 oz.	381
Cabbage (steamed), 1 cup	50	Spinach (steamed), 1 cup	244
Cauliflower (steamed), 1 cup	34	Soybeans, 1 cup	73
Collards (steamed), 1 cup	152	Soymilk (fortified), 1 cup	150
Corn Tortilla, 1	60	Tofu (firm), 1/2 cup	258
Cornbread, 1 piece	28	Turnip greens, 1 cup	198
Figs, 5 medium	135	Whole wheat bread, 1 slice	17

Sources: *Back to Eden,* Jethro Kloss; *Health Nutrient Bible,* Lynne Sonberg; website: *www.ucsfhealth.org/adult/edu/calciumContent/index.html*

(Phosphorus) combines with calcium and vitamins A and D in proper proportion for balanced bone structure and body metabolism. Natural sources include, all organ meats; fish and cod-liver oil; natural cheese; soybeans, raw spinach, cucumbers, alfalfa sprouts, peas, kale, mustard greens, watercress; brazil nuts; whole-grain rye, whole wheat, bran; and raw wheat germ.

(Magnesium) is necessary for calcium and vitamin D metabolism which helps to build and prevent the softening of bones. Natural sources are string beans, peas, garbanzos, kidney beans, dried lima beans; Brussels sprouts, chard, cucumbers, alfalfa sprouts, raw spinach; bran and whole wheat; avocados; pine nuts and sunflower seeds; prunes and raisins; and honey.

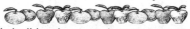

Thy food shall be thy remedy. – Hippocrates, 400 BC

Manganese is an important trace mineral that serves as a carrier of oxygen from the blood to the cells. It is particularly important in the nourishment of the intervertebral disks and cartilage that have no direct blood circulation.

Natural Manganese Sources include fish, poultry, liver, fertile egg yolk, organ meats, all natural cheese; agar, dulse, kelp; potatoes, especially the skins (steam or bake in jackets and eat the skins); lettuce, watercress, celery, onions; alfalfa sprouts, peas, all beans; bran and organic cornmeal; almonds, filberts, chestnuts, walnuts (the best); and bananas.

Remember that your body must have natural organic minerals (i.e., from plants and living sources). Neither humans or even animals can assimilate inorganic rock minerals, as they come directly from earth. Only plants can digest inorganic minerals into an organic form that can be used by animals and humans.

So, if you take mineral supplements, make sure these are from organic sources. To take inorganic calcium tablets, for example, would not supply your bones with the calcium they need; it would only clog up your system with indigestible chalk. Health Stores have natural supplementary organic sources of calcium and other organic minerals essential for strong, healthy bones.

Vitamins Essential to a Healthy Spine

All the natural vitamins are important for health. Of special importance to a healthy spine are vitamins A, C and D for building and maintaining strong, resilient bone structure. The B-complex vitamins are essential to the spinal cord and nervous system.

Vitamins A & D are essential in regulating the use of calcium and phosphorus – the two major elements in the formation, building and maintenance of bones – in the body. Vitamins A and D are also vital to the efficient functioning of the nervous system. They act together as catalysts in this all-important phase of body metabolism. Without them, the parathyroid glands of the endocrine system cannot carry out their primary function of maintaining the balanced interaction and distribution of calcium and phosphorus, and both bones and nerves deteriorate. There is a marked drop in bone density in people whose diet has been deficient in vitamins A and D over a period of time. Abnormal spaces appear in the bone structure, and the bone cells become thin, brittle, and almost looks like swiss cheese: this is osteoporosis.

(Natural sources of vitamin A) are colored fruits and vegetables such as carrots, yams, yellow squash, papaya, apricots, peaches, melons and dairy products (we avoid), fertile eggs, liver, fish and cod liver oil (contains A & D).

(Natural sources of vitamin D) also include fish liver oils, unsaturated fats, fresh fertile eggs, organic milk and butter, but the prime source is sunshine. A daily gentle sunbath (before 10am or after 3pm) will supply your quota of vitamin D, as well as improve your health in many other ways. Give your body time to absorb vitamin D through the skin before washing off perspiration after a sunbath.

(Vitamin C) supplies collagen, the adhesive that holds together all the cells in the bones and nerves and body tissues. Without C, we would literally fall apart. Since the body does not store this powerful antioxidant, we need a constant supply of vitamin C in the daily diet.

(Natural sources of C) are citrus fruits, berries, greens, cabbage and green bell peppers. These should be eaten raw and fresh, since cooking easily destroys vitamin C.

B-COMPLEX VITAMINS:

(Vitamin B1:) Thiamin chloride – often called the anti-neuritic or anti-beriberi vitamin – aids growth and digestion and is essential for normal functioning of nerve tissues, muscles and heart. Deficiency signs include nervous irritability, fatigue, insomnia, loss of weight and appetite, weakness and lassitude and mental depression.

(Vitamin B2:) Riboflavin, or vitamin G, promotes general health and particularly affects health of the eyes, mouth and skin. Deficiency is often evidenced by itching, burning or bloodshot eyes, inflammation of the mouth, purplish tongue and cracking of mouth corners.

(Vitamin B6:) Pyridoxine prevents various nervous and skin disorders. It aids food assimilation, protein and fat metabolism. Nervousness, insomnia, skin eruption and loss of muscular control are signs of deficiency.

Vitamin B12: Cobalamin, the *great energy vitamin*, aids in important formation and regeneration of red blood cells (produced in bone marrow) and is essential in prevention of anemia, osteoporosis and heart disease. It also promotes growth in children, and is a tonic for adults, especially seniors! Deficiency may lead to pernicious anemia, growth failure and poor appetite in children and seniors and the above diseases. (See web: *www.homocysteine.com*)

Natural sources of B-complex vitamins: It's important to include the entire B-complex in your diet, and Nature has provided for this. Bragg Nutritional Yeast heads the B-rich foods list, followed by raw wheat germ and beef, liver, both fresh and dehydrated. Other organ meats, especially beef heart and brains and lamb kidney, are rich B-complex sources, as well as fertile eggs, especially the yolk; fish; and natural cheeses. Natural, unsalted peanut butter (not hydrogenated) is an excellent source of B-complex vitamins; so are raw or freshly roasted peanuts. Whole grains such as barley and 100% whole-grain flours such as buckwheat flour, cornmeal, etc., are included, as well as organic oatmeal and rice husks. Vegetable sources include raw and dried beans like lima, soybeans and green beans; raw and dried green peas; and leafy vegetables such as collards, turnip greens, mustard greens, spinach, broccoli and cabbage. B-rich fruits are oranges, grapefruit, bananas, avocados and cantaloupe. Blackstrap molasses is a fine source. Alone or with other dishes, mushrooms add B-vitamins.

97

We take natural vitamins and mineral supplements – it's added insurance for super health. Be sure they are from organic, all natural sources – the best for your health.

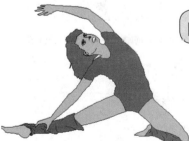

Body and Mind Work Together

Whatever occurs in the mind affects the body and vice versa. The mind and the body cannot be considered independently. When the two are out of sync, then both emotional and physical stress can erupt.
– Hippocrates, Father of Medicine, 400 BC

As I stride along on my daily 2 to 4 mile brisk walk with hand weights that help keep my bones strong, I say to myself, often out loud, Health, Strength, Youth, Vitality, Joy, Peace and Salvation for Eternity! – Patricia Bragg

Don't Stiffen and Age Your Joints

Nutrition is as important as exercise for a strong, supple spine. Even the Spine Motion Exercises cannot achieve permanent efficacy if you allow vertebral joints to stiffen and calcify with inorganic minerals and toxic acid crystals from improper eating or drinking.

As noted, the average civilized diet is highly acidic in content, upsetting the natural alkaline-acid balance. After each meal, an indigestible, toxic residue remains, which takes the form of toxic acid crystals, inorganic calcium-like mineral substances that cannot be absorbed by the body. So where do these toxic acid crystals go?

Remember, the movable joints of the skeletal system, including those of the spinal column, are lubricated with synovial fluid which, under normal conditions, is ample to last a lifetime. However, this space between the joints offers the easiest location for deposits of the indigestible buildup of toxic acid crystals. Gradually, the synovial fluid is displaced by these calcified substances and the joints start becoming stiff and painful. Movable joints are one place where you don't want calcium, especially inorganic calcium, which replaces the vital lubricating synovial fluid with a kind of toxic crystalline cement.

The intervertebral disks are also subject to this type of painful calcification. This is one of the main reasons why it's important for you to follow the Basic Rules of Natural Nutrition that we have outlined for you. If you plan your menus along these lines, you will maintain a diet with the proper alkaline-acid balance (which is about $3/5$ alkaline and $2/5$ acid). In general, fruits and vegetables (with a few exceptions) are alkaline forming, while proteins, starches, fats and sugars are acid forming.

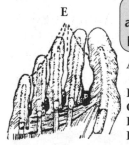

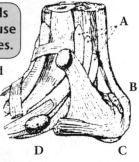

Deposits of Inorganic Minerals and Toxic Acid Crystals can cause pain in Heels and Between Toes.

A. Inorganic minerals deposited under the tendons.
B. Under the Achilles' tendon.
C. Under the heel.
D. Under the middle foot.
E. Between Toes.

Pure Water is Essential For Health!

Yes, pure water is essential for health. You get it from the natural juices of vegetables, fruits and other foods, or from the water of high purity obtained by steam distillation which is the best method. Another effective method combines de-ionization and purification.

The body is constantly working for you, breaking down old bone and tissue cells and replacing them with new ones. As the body casts off the old minerals and other products of broken-down cells it must obtain new supplies of the essential elements for the new cells. Scientists are beginning to understand that various kinds of dental problems, many types of arthritis and some forms of hardening of the arteries are due to imbalances in the body's levels of calcium, phosphorus and magnesium. Disorders can also be caused by imbalances in the ratios of various minerals to each other.

Each healthy body requires a proper balance within itself of all the nutritive elements. It is just as bad for any individual to have too much of one item as it is to have too little of that one or of another one. It takes appropriate levels of phosphorus and magnesium to keep calcium in solution so it can be formed into new bone and teeth. Yet, there must not be too much of those nor too little calcium in the diet, or old bone will be taken away but new bone will not be formed.

In addition, we now know that diets which are unbalanced and inappropriate for a given individual can deplete the body of calcium, magnesium, potassium, and other major and minor elements. Diets which are high in meats, fish, eggs and grains or their products may provide unbalanced excesses of phosphorus. This will deplete calcium and magnesium from the bones and tissues of the body and cause them to be lost in the urine. A diet high in fats will tend to increase the uptake of phosphorus from the intestines relative to calcium and other basic minerals. Such a high-fat diet can produce losses of calcium, magnesium, and other basic minerals as a high-phosphorus diet does.

99

Pure water is the best drink for a wise man. – Henry David Thoreau

Fluorine is a Deadly Poison!

Millions of innocent people have been brainwashed by the aluminum companies to erroneously believe that adding toxic sodium fluoride (their waste by-product) to our drinking water will reduce tooth decay in our children. Americans get sodium fluoride in their drinking water without thinking about it. A chemical cousin of sodium, fluorine in high doses is used as a rat and roach killer and as a deadly pesticide.

Yet this deadly sodium fluoride, injected virtually by government edict into drinking water in the proportion of 1.2 parts per million (PPM), has been declared by the US Public Health Service to be "safe for all human consumption." Every chemist knows that such "absolute safety" is not only unattainable, but a total illusion!

Keep Toxic Fluoride Out of Water & Foods!

Most water Americans drink has fluoride in it, including tap, bottled and canned drinks and foods, plus in most toothpastes! Now, the *American Dental Association* is insisting the FDA mandate the addition of fluoride to all bottled waters! Defend your right to drink pure, non-fluoridated tap and bottled waters! Challenge and please help stop all local and state water fluoridation policies! Call, write, fax or e-mail all state officials and Congresspeople (see web: *www.firstgov.gov*) and send them a copy of our water book.

These 11 Associations Stopped Endorsing Water Fluoridation Way Back in 1996

- American Heart Association
- American Cancer Society
- American Diabetes Assoc.
- American Chiropractic Assoc.
- National Kidney Foundation
- American Academy of Allergy & Immunology
- Chronic Fatigue Syndrome Action Network
- National Institute of Law Municipal Officers
- American Civil Liberties Union • Soc. of Toxicology
- American Psychiatric Association

Check the Following Websites for Fluoride Updates:

- www.fluorideresearch.org
- www.keepers-of-the-well.org
- www.tldp.com/fluoride.htm
- www.bruha.com/fluoride/
- www.slweb.org/bibliography.html
- www.fluoridealert.org
- www.fluoridation.com
- www.citizens.org
- www.gjne.com/cfsdwh
- www.bragg.com

Ten Common Sense Reasons Why You Should Only Drink Pure, Distilled Water!

- There are over 12,000 toxic chemicals on the market today . . . and 500 more are being added yearly! Wherever you live, in the city or on the farm, some of these chemicals are getting into your drinking water. Beware of chemicalized water.

- No one on the face of the earth today knows what effect these chemicals could have upon the body as they blend into thousands of different combinations. It is like making a mixture of colors; one drop could change the color.

- Proper equipment hasn't been designed yet to detect some of these chemicals and may not be for many years to come.

- The body is made up of approximately 70% water. Therefore, don't you think you should be particular about the type of water you drink?

- The Navy has been drinking distilled water for years!

- Distilled water is chemical and mineral free. Distillation removes all the chemicals and impurities from water that are possible to remove. If distillation doesn't remove them, there is no known method today that will.

- The body does need minerals . . . but it is not necessary that they come from water. There is not one mineral in water which cannot be found more abundantly in food! Water is the most unreliable source of minerals because it varies from one area to another. The food we eat – not the water we drink – is the best source of organic minerals!

- Distilled water is used for intravenous feeding, inhalation therapy, prescriptions and baby formulas. Therefore, doesn't it make common sense that it is good for everyone?

- Thousands of water distillers have been sold throughout the United States and around the world to individuals, families, dentists, doctors, hospitals, nursing homes and government agencies, and these informed, alert consumers are helping protect their health by using only steam distilled water. They don't want toxic chemicals.

- With chemicals, pollutants and impurities in our water, it makes good sense to clean up the water you drink, using Mother Nature's inexpensive way – distillation.

101

BRAGGZYME®

SUPERIOR SYSTEMIC ENZYMES
Support for joints, muscles and immune system
FOR HEALTHY ACTIVE LIFESTYLE AND HEART SUPPORT

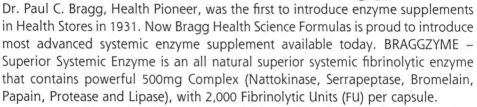

Dr. Paul C. Bragg, Health Pioneer, was the first to introduce enzyme supplements in Health Stores in 1931. Now Bragg Health Science Formulas is proud to introduce most advanced systemic enzyme supplement available today. BRAGGZYME – Superior Systemic Enzyme is an all natural superior systemic fibrinolytic enzyme that contains powerful 500mg Complex (Nattokinase, Serrapeptase, Bromelain, Papain, Protease and Lipase), with 2,000 Fibrinolytic Units (FU) per capsule.

"Good Circulation is Key to A Healthy Body!" — Paul C. Bragg, ND, PhD.

This exclusive systemic enzyme blend provides nutritional and cardiovascular support you need to maintain healthy fibrin levels to avoid dangerous blood clots in the circulatory system.* Braggzyme helps fight inflammation and helps to maintain normal inflammatory response for over-all health.*

- Enzyme support for back, joint, muscle, tendon and immune health system.*
- Boost energy levels – infuses life-giving oxygen to every cell in your body.*
- Nutritional support to help maintain a normal inflammatory response.*
- Helps eliminate dangerous fibrin levels for a healthier blood flow.*
- Helps keep your hands, feet and the entire body warm.*
- Helps improve and keep memory and brain sharp.*
- Contains no animal derivatives, no yeast, no wheat, no artificial flavors and no artificial colors.
- Kosher Certified
- 100% Safe, All Natural Veg. Formula in Veg. Cap

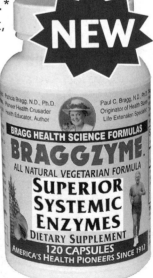

NEW

> *These statements have not been evaluated by the Food and Drug Administration. This product is not intended to diagnose, treat, cure, or prevent any disease.

"I have been taking Braggzyme for the last several months, and have felt a major improvement in my knee pain caused by sports, snowboarding, etc. Thanks, Braggzyme!"
– Brian Evans, Manager, Lassens Natural Foods, Santa Barbara, CA

My doctor said that elevated fibrinogen levels are associated with an increased risk of heart attack and strokes because it can promote formation of dangerous blood clots. Good news! I've been taking Braggzyme and my blood fibrinogen level was 329 and it came down 50 points, now it's a safe 279.
– Kathy Duerr, Portland, OR

Since I have been on Braggzyme, I have tremendous energy and now have absolutely no more aches and pains! My memory is sharper and I am enjoying my vibrant energy. Thanks to Braggzyme. – Robert De Castro, Newport Beach, CA

Chapter 10

Put Your Back into It!

Use Your "Backbone" for Physical Fitness

In carrying out this Program of Physical Fitness with Spine Motion, you must use your backbone, in both senses of the word! In the folklore sense, of courage and willpower, you must use your backbone to transform your pattern of life from one of merely tolerable existence to living in the full joy of radiant health! Particularly in the beginning, you will need mental discipline and will power to reprogram your lifestyle habits of diet, posture and physical exercise in accordance with the Natural Laws of Health and Fitness, we have outlined for you.

Vital in this transformation is the exercise of your backbone: stretching and strengthening your spinal column with these unique Bragg Spine Motion Exercises, and the easy-to-do Posture and Back Strengthening Exercises. Faithfully follow instructions we have given you.

103

Do the exercises in this book slowly and gently for first week or so. At first, feel your way along so as not to get your muscles sore with overly vigorous contractions. Always exercise short of the point of pain. No matter what, don't stop your daily routine! A slight soreness is natural when your muscles have been unused, but it will disappear when you continue your program.

Remember: if you can move a muscle, you can strengthen it. We have never seen anyone who could move a muscle and was willing to really exercise daily yet couldn't develop a limber and supple spine, gain added strength, have a more active life, look and feel better and get more real enjoyment out of daily living.

Never forget: if you don't use your spine, you will lose it. It will become prematurely old, stiff and painful. The body and spine remain youthful, supple and strong only with sufficient use, exercise and healthy living!

The journal Circulation *reports people who don't make efforts to exercise, face the same risk of heart disease as people who smoke a pack of cigarettes daily.*

You Are as Young or Old as Your Spine Is

No matter how you have neglected and abused your spine, by following the instructions given in this book, you can reverse the condition. The recuperative powers of the human body are tremendous. The body is a self-repairing and self-healing miracle. You must give your body the natural health aids it needs. When the correct nutrition and exercise are provided, you help your spine repair and restore itself to health.

Let us repeat: the body remains strong only if it is used. More than 70% of the patients in physicians' offices today have under-exercised spines. Your body and your spine need daily exercise and good posture habits!

Make Spine Motion Exercises a part of your morning routine, like brushing your teeth or combing your hair Don't tell us you *"don't have time"* to have a limber spine and a physically fit body! That's absolute nonsense. If you have a sense of true values, you will find the time to take care of your precious body. It's the only one you'll ever get, so take extra special care of it! It will reward you with a bright and healthy life. *Get started now!*

Within a few weeks of following the Bragg Spine Motion Program outlined, your spine will feel more flexible and supple. You will walk with a spring in your step. You will feel the vital energy surging through your body. You will be surprised how wonderful you feel when your spine limbers up! You will find that you do not tire as easily. You will have more go-power and energetic drive.

It will not stop there. Each day, you will add new zest, vigor and power to your body. Remember: the world is alive, and you're alive; you are never too old to feel youthful and enjoy an ageless powerful body! Now, get started and really begin to feel fully alive again! Like thousands of others, you will get a new lease on life as you follow The Bragg Healthy Lifestyle with this Back Fitness Program with Spine Motion. Life is a real joy to enjoy when your spine and body functions perfectly.

The human body has one ability not possessed by any machine, the ability to repair and heal itself. – George E. Crile, Jr. M.D.

Exercise and Eat for Total Health and Fitness

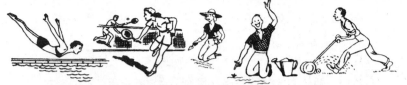

The Bragg Healthy Lifestyle
For a Lifetime of Super Health

In a broad sense, "The Bragg Healthy Lifestyle for the Total Person" is a combination of physical, mental, emotional, social and spiritual components. The ability of the individual to function effectively in his environment depends on how smoothly these components function as a whole. Of all the qualities that comprise an integrated personality, a totally healthy, fit body is one of the most desirable . . . so start today for achieving your health goals!

A person may be said to be totally physically fit if he functions as a total personality with efficiency and without pain or discomfort of any kind. This is to have a Painless, Tireless, Ageless body, possessing sufficient muscular strength and endurance to maintain a healthy posture and successfully carry on the duties imposed by life and the environment, to meet emergencies satisfactorily and have enough energy for recreation and social obligations after the "work day" has ended. It is to meet the requirements of his environment through possessing the resilience to recover rapidly from fatigue, tension, stress and strain of daily living without the aid of stimulants, drugs or alcohol, and enjoy natural recharging sleep at night and awaken fit and alert in the morning for the challenges of the new fresh day ahead.

Keeping the body totally healthy and fit is not a job for the uninformed or the careless person. It requires an understanding of the body and of a healthy lifestyle and then following it for a long, happy lifetime of health! The result of "The Bragg Healthy Lifestyle" is to wake up the possibilities within you, rejuvenate your body, mind and soul to total balanced health. It's within your reach, so don't procrastinate, start today! Our hearts go out to touch your heart with nourishing, caring love for your total health and life!

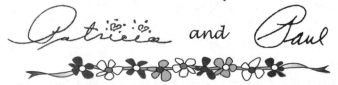

Patricia and *Paul*

Dear friend, I wish above all things that thou may prosper and be in health, even as the soul prospers. – 3 John 2

105

Dr. James Balch's Helpful Suggestions for Dealing with Back Pain

Nearly 80% of adults deal with back pain some time in their lives. Aside from ruptured disks, backache may result from muscle strain, build-up of acidic byproducts, stress, poor posture, calcium deficiency, kidney, bladder and prostate problems, etc. There are many causes for back pain as there are healthy alternatives. In his popular guidebook *Prescription for Nutritional Healing**
Dr. James Balch gives simple, healthful suggestions.

Dr. Balch's Helpful suggestions for Back Pain:

- Avoid meats and animal protein products until you are healed, as they contain uric acid which puts undue strain on the kidneys that contributes to back pain. Eat no gravies, fats, sugar, refined processed foods.

- Follow a fasting program faithfully: one day a week.

- When pain hits, immediately drink two large glasses of distilled water, as pains are frequently connected to dehydration! The body needs at least eight 8-ounce glasses of water a day to flush out toxins and acidic wastes that builds up in your muscles and tissues.

- If pain follows an injury or sudden movement, apply ice on & off first 48 hours, then heat. Rest on firm bed.

- To relieve muscle back pain, take warm bath or apply (on & off) heating pad. Capsaicin, Arnica salve, & DMSO helps.

- Once acute pain and inflammation has subsided, do gentle exercises to strengthen abdominal muscles in order to prevent recurrences. Gentle half sit-ups help this.

- When carrying hand bags, etc. on shoulder, switch the weight to the other shoulder from time to time.

- Learn to reduce any body stress. Practice relaxation techniques such as walking, deep slow breathing, meditation and gentle yoga.

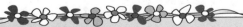

Bragg Health Books were My Conversion to The Healthy Way.
– James Balch, M.D., Co Author *Prescription for Nutritional Healing*

More of Dr. Balch's Help With Back Pain

- Wear comfortable, well-made shoes. Caution: the higher the heels of your shoes, the more risk of backache!

- Move around. Don't stay in same position for long periods.

- Never lean forward without bending your knees. Lift with your legs, arms and abdomen, not with your back. Avoid lifting anything heavier than twenty pounds. To work near the ground, squat rather than bending at the waist.

- Always push large objects rather than pulling them.

- It's best to sleep on your back, not on your stomach. Sleep on a firm mattress with your head elevated on a pillow, and some like a small pillow under their knees.

- Maintain healthy weight and get regular moderate exercise. Activities good for back include swimming, exercycle or biking, walking, rowing, stretching and gentle yoga.

- If pain lasts longer than seventy-two hours, radiates into the legs, includes numbness, or is accompanied by an unexplained weight loss, consult your health care provider.

- If you have pain on one side in small of back and feel sick, and if you have a fever, see your doctor or Med Center immediately. You may have a kidney infection.

- If pain follows an injury and is accompanied by sudden loss of bladder or bowel control, if you have difficulty moving any limb, or if you feel numbness, pain, or tingling in a limb, do not move, but call for medical help immediately. You may have hurt your spinal cord.

– Dr. James Balch, Co-Author of *Prescription for Nutritional Healing.*
*Available in Health Stores and Book Stores

Caring hands have healing life-force energy. All ages, even babies to family pets thrive on daily loving, soothing, healing touching and massages. Everyone benefits from healing massages and treatments! – Patricia Bragg

Having heard the word, keep it, and bring forth fruit with patience. – Luke 8:15

PILATES, a complex gentle form of exercises – a fusion of western and eastern philosophies, teaches you about breathing with movement, body mechanics, balance, co-ordination, positioning of body, spatial awareness, muscle strength and flexibility. – www.pilates-studio.com

Types of Vertebrae

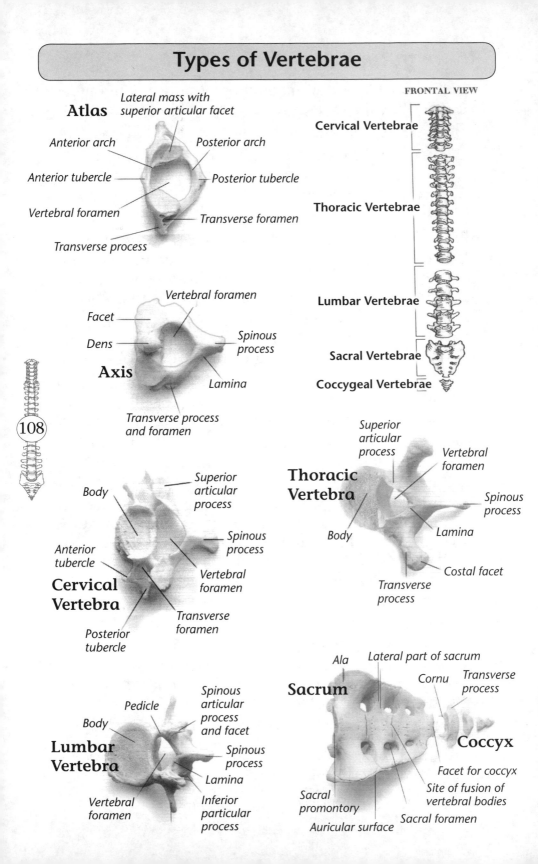

FRONTAL VIEW

Cervical Vertebrae

Thoracic Vertebrae

Lumbar Vertebrae

Sacral Vertebrae

Coccygeal Vertebrae

Atlas

Lateral mass with superior articular facet

Anterior arch

Posterior arch

Anterior tubercle

Posterior tubercle

Vertebral foramen

Transverse foramen

Transverse process

Axis

Vertebral foramen

Facet

Dens

Spinous process

Lamina

Transverse process and foramen

Cervical Vertebra

Body

Superior articular process

Spinous process

Anterior tubercle

Vertebral foramen

Posterior tubercle

Transverse foramen

Thoracic Vertebra

Superior articular process

Vertebral foramen

Spinous process

Body

Lamina

Costal facet

Transverse process

Lumbar Vertebra

Pedicle

Spinous articular process and facet

Body

Spinous process

Lamina

Inferior particular process

Vertebral foramen

Sacrum

Ala

Lateral part of sacrum

Cornu

Transverse process

Coccyx

Facet for coccyx

Site of fusion of vertebral bodies

Sacral promontory

Sacral foramen

Auricular surface

The Back Pain Epidemic

The back and spinal system are so complex that it's often difficult to pinpoint the exact cause of the back pain (*researchers have found strong link between sedentary lifestyle and weak stomach/back muscles and chronic back pain*). Add to this the many different approaches to understanding what is wrong, as well as the variety of options for addressing back problems, and you have a whole wide world revolving around the common experience of back pain felt worldwide.

This is true in America, where there is so much variety available in back treatments (see pages 117-120). The less industrialized countries often have fewer patient complaints about back pain – not because people don't suffer from it, but because it's considered part of life and they are not aware of it as a specific medical condition that can be diagnosed and cured. In contrast, backaches are the second most common reason for doctor visits in the United States (cold and flu are first). And for all the available treatments for Americans, they are generally dissatisfied with the medical care they receive. *When something hurts, we want it fixed – and fast*, says Bill McCarberg, Director of Pain Services at Kaiser Permanente in San Diego, *It's very frustrating to visit the doctor and find out that, in most cases, the doctor can't solve the problem.*

109

In spite of the difficulty in pinpointing the cause and best treatment of back problems, years of research and experience have lead the medical community to some sure knowledge: *I think we can say with certainty now that bed rest and traction are a bad idea*, says Daniel Cherkin, a scientific investigator at the Center for Health Studies. *They both can weaken muscles supporting the back and make the problems worse.* Most researchers also agree that only between 2% to 5% of back patients really require surgery, and only for cases of tumors, spinal fractures, and extreme leg pain due to nerve compression in spine. Beyond these, it's up to each individual to seek and discover approach that works best for them! For this reason, be familiar with alternative therapies, Chiropractic, Acupuncture, Acupressure, Exercise, etc., listed in this book.

Exercise: Some is good, often more is better. – New England Journal of Medicine

Spinal Column – Your Vital Connection

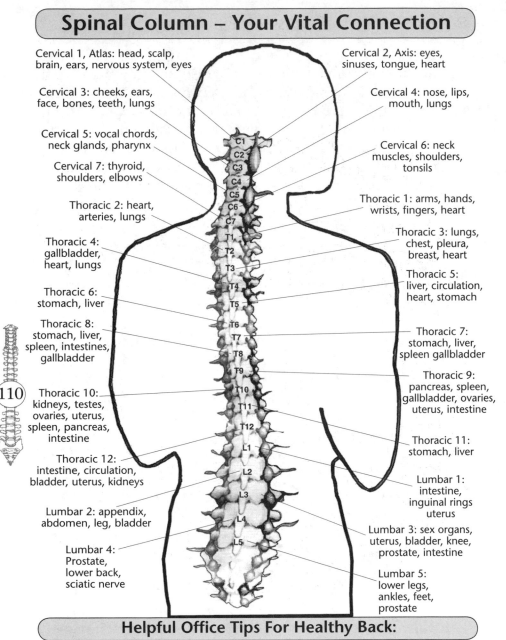

Cervical 1, Atlas: head, scalp, brain, ears, nervous system, eyes

Cervical 2, Axis: eyes, sinuses, tongue, heart

Cervical 3: cheeks, ears, face, bones, teeth, lungs

Cervical 4: nose, lips, mouth, lungs

Cervical 5: vocal chords, neck glands, pharynx

Cervical 6: neck muscles, shoulders, tonsils

Cervical 7: thyroid, shoulders, elbows

Thoracic 1: arms, hands, wrists, fingers, heart

Thoracic 2: heart, arteries, lungs

Thoracic 3: lungs, chest, pleura, breast, heart

Thoracic 4: gallbladder, heart, lungs

Thoracic 5: liver, circulation, heart, stomach

Thoracic 6: stomach, liver

Thoracic 7: stomach, liver, spleen gallbladder

Thoracic 8: stomach, liver, spleen, intestines, gallbladder

Thoracic 9: pancreas, spleen, gallbladder, ovaries, uterus, intestine

Thoracic 10: kidneys, testes, ovaries, uterus, spleen, pancreas, intestine

Thoracic 11: stomach, liver

Thoracic 12: intestine, circulation, bladder, uterus, kidneys

Lumbar 1: intestine, inguinal rings uterus

Lumbar 2: appendix, abdomen, leg, bladder

Lumbar 3: sex organs, uterus, bladder, knee, prostate, intestine

Lumbar 4: Prostate, lower back, sciatic nerve

Lumbar 5: lower legs, ankles, feet, prostate

C1 C2 C3 C4 C5 C6 C7 T1 T2 T3 T4 T5 T6 T7 T8 T9 T10 T11 T12 L1 L2 L3 L4 L5

110

Helpful Office Tips For Healthy Back:

- Change chair height so your forearms are level with desk and hands at keyboard level are best.
- Use headset or speaker phone if you have significant phone use. This benefits you by reducing muscle tension in neck and back.
- Change your position at least every 20 minutes. If you stay active – without overdoing things, you will protect your back and may alleviate any back symptoms. (See web: *spineuniverse.com*)
- Don't ever sit with your legs crossed.

We must always change, renew, rejuvenate; otherwise, we harden. – Goethe

Reflexology – Pressure Points for your Feet

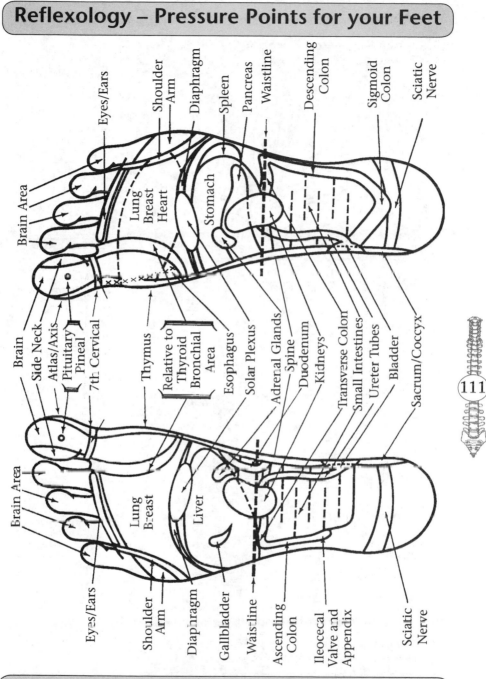

Eyes/Ears · Shoulder Arm · Diaphragm · Spleen · Pancreas · Waistline · Descending Colon · Sigmoid Colon · Sciatic Nerve

Brain Area

Lung Breast Heart · Stomach

Brain · Side Neck · Atlas/Axis · Pituitary Pineal · 7th Cervical · Thymus · Relative to Thyroid Bronchial Area · Esophagus · Solar Plexus · Adrenal Glands · Spine · Duodenum · Kidneys · Transverse Colon · Small Intestines · Ureter Tubes · Bladder · Sacrum/Coccyx

111

Brain Area

Lung Breast · Liver

Eyes/Ears · Shoulder Arm · Diaphragm · Gallbladder · Waistline · Ascending Colon · Ileocecal Valve and Appendix · Sciatic Nerve

REFLEXOLOGY AND ZONE THERAPY

Founded by Eunice Ingham, author of *The Story The Feet Can Tell*, who was inspired by a Bragg Health Crusade when she was 17. Reflexology helps the body by removing crystalline deposits from meridians (nerve endings) of the feet through deep pressure massage. It helps activate body's flow of healthy energy by dislodging any collected deposits around nerve endings. (Chart by Eunice Ingham's nephew Dwight Byers.) Web: reflexology-usa.net

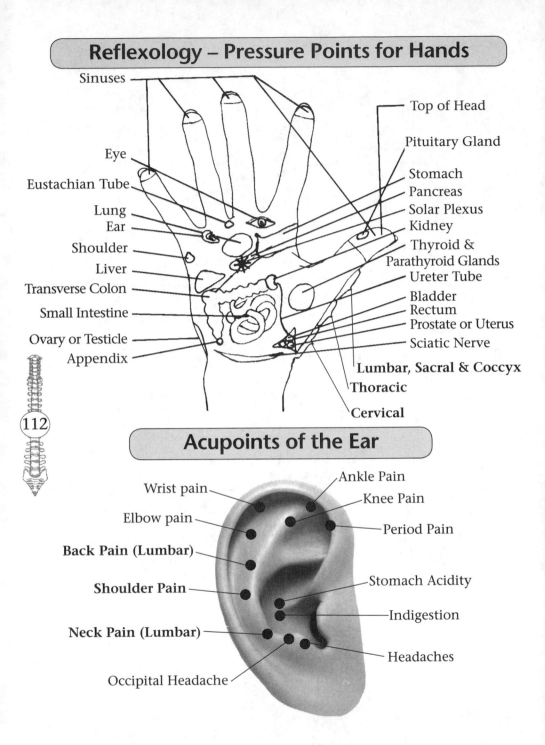

Reflexology – Pressure Points for Hands

Sinuses
Eye
Eustachian Tube
Lung
Ear
Shoulder
Liver
Transverse Colon
Small Intestine
Ovary or Testicle
Appendix

Top of Head
Pituitary Gland
Stomach
Pancreas
Solar Plexus
Kidney
Thyroid & Parathyroid Glands
Ureter Tube
Bladder
Rectum
Prostate or Uterus
Sciatic Nerve
Lumbar, Sacral & Coccyx
Thoracic
Cervical

112

Acupoints of the Ear

Wrist pain
Elbow pain
Back Pain (Lumbar)
Shoulder Pain
Neck Pain (Lumbar)
Occipital Headache

Ankle Pain
Knee Pain
Period Pain
Stomach Acidity
Indigestion
Headaches

Apply strong pressure using index finger and thumb (place thumb at back of ear). Squeeze point for about two minutes, then massage (I do this nightly). You can repeat this throughout the day whenever convenient (acupressure ear points are bilateral – same on both ears). Ear points respond well to acupressure and can be combined with other body acupressure points or used by themselves.

Acupoints of the Spine

These are special acupoints located on the back that help balance the body and also promote wellness.

Circulation Sex

Gallbladder

Stomach

Kidney

Large Intestine

Urinary Bladder

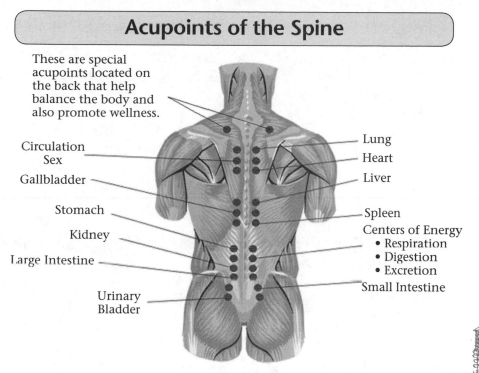

Lung
Heart
Liver

Spleen
Centers of Energy
• Respiration
• Digestion
• Excretion
Small Intestine

Design created by David Carmos, Ph.D. from *The Acupoint Book* and *You're Never Too Old To Become Young* by David Carmos, Ph.D. and Shawn Miller, D.C. (See Web: www.perfecthealthnow.com)

What is Acupressure?

Acupressure Potent Points is an ancient healing art that uses fingers to press key local points on skin's surface to stimulate body's natural self-curative inner healing abilities. When these points are pressed, they release muscular tension reaching also to the body's trigger points to promote healthier blood circulation and increase the vital life force to aid healing. Acupressure is the most effective method for self-treatment of tension-related ailments by using the power and sensitivity of the touch of the human hand. See web: *www.acupressure.com*

How Acupressure Can Help Relieve Pain

One of the popular alternative therapies available to help relieve back pain is acupressure, which is often described as acupuncture without needles. Acupressure is a system of massage that promotes the life energy, stimulating meridian points whether needles or fingers are used.

Acupressure You Can Do Yourself

Foremost among the advantages of acupressure's healing touch is that it's safe to do on yourself and others – even if you've never done it before – just follow the instructions and go gently and slowly. There are no side effects from drugs and the only equipment needed are your own two hands. You can practice acupressure therapy any time, anywhere on friends, family and yourself! The acupressure points are areas on the body that are sensitive to the body's bioelectrical impulses. When you stimulate these points, it triggers the release of natural endorphins. As a result, pain is blocked and the flow of blood and oxygen to the affected area is increased. This causes the muscles to relax and promotes healing.

Besides relieving pain, the acupressure can help rebalance the body by dissolving the tensions and stresses that keep the body from functioning smoothly and which inhibit the immune system. Troublemaking tension tends to concentrate around acupressure points. Along with Acupressure, you can use a combination of the self-help methods given in this book that can help improve your overall health and you will feel more alive, healthy, and in harmony with your life. *With our love and blessings,*

Patricia and *Paul*

Morning Resolve To Start Your Day

I will this day live a simple, sincere and serene life; repelling promptly every thought of impurity, discontent, anxiety, discouragement and fear. I will cultivate health, cheerfulness, happiness, charity and the love of brotherhood; exercising economy in expenditure, generosity in giving, carefulness in conversation and diligence in appointed service. I pledge fidelity to every trust and a childlike faith in God. In particular, I will be faithful in those habits of prayer, study, work, nutrition, physical exercise, deep breathing and good posture. I shall fast for a 24 hour period each week, eat only healthy foods and get sufficient sleep each night. I will make every effort to improve myself physically, mentally, emotionally and spiritually every day.

Morning Prayer used by Patricia Bragg and her father, Paul C. Bragg

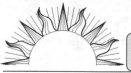

MY DAILY HEALTH JOURNAL

Today is:___/___/___

> *I have said my morning resolve and am ready to practice*
> *The Bragg Healthy Lifestyle today and every day.*

Yesterday I went to bed at:　　　Today I arose at:　　　Weight:

Today I practiced the No-Heavy Breakfast or No-Breakfast Plan: ☐ yes ☐ no

• For Breakfast I drank:　　　　　　　　　　　Time:

　For Breakfast I ate:

　　　　　　　　　　　　　　　　　　　　　Time:

　Supplements:

• For Lunch I ate:　　　　　　　　　　　　Time:

　Supplements:

• For Dinner I ate:　　　　　　　　　　　　Time:

　Supplements:

• _____Glasses of Water I Drank during the Day

　List Snacks – Kind and When:

• I took part in these physical (walking, gym, etc.) activities today:

Grade each on scale of 1 to 10 (desired optimum health is 10).
• I rate my day for the following categories:

Previous Night's Sleep:	Stress/Anxiety:
Energy Level:	Elimination:
Physical Activity, Exercise:	Health:
Peacefulness:	Accomplishments:
Happiness:	Self-Esteem:

• General Comments, Reactions and To Do List:

Mother Nature
Loves You To
Enjoy Her Beauty

116

Let me look upward
into the branches
Of the towering oak
And know that it grew
slowly and well.

Give me, amidst
the confusion
of my day
The calmness of the
everlasting hills.

Let me pause
to look at a flower,
to smell a rose —
God's autograph,
to chat with a friend,
to read a few lines
from a good book.

Break the tensions
of my nerves
With the soothing music
of singing streams
and gentle rains
That live in
my memory.

Follow steps of the Godly,
and stay on the right path
to enjoy life to the fullest.

– Proverbs 2:20-21

Mother Nature and friendship are cozy shelters for life's rainy days.

Chapter 11

Healthy Alternative Therapies and Massage Techniques

Try Them – They Work Miracles!

Explore these wonderful natural methods of healing your body. Finally over 600 Medical Schools in the U.S. are teaching Healthy Alternative Therapies. Please check out the websites. Now choose the best healing techniques for you:

ACUPUNCTURE/ACUPRESSURE Acupuncture directs and rechannels body energy by inserting hair-thin needles (*use only disposable needles*) at specific points on the body. It's used for pain, backaches, migraines and general health and body dysfunctions. Used in Asia for centuries, acupuncture is safe, virtually painless and has no side effects. **Acupressure** is based on the same principles and uses finger pressure and massage rather than needles. Websites offer info, check them out. Web: *acupuncturetoday.com*

CHIROPRACTIC Chiropractic was founded in Davenport, Iowa in 1885 by Daniel David Palmer. There are now many schools in the U.S., and graduates are joining Health Practitioners in all nations of the world to share healing techniques. Chiropractic is popular, is the largest U.S. healing profession benefitting literally millions. Treatment involves soft tissue, spinal and body adjustment to free the nervous system of interferences with normal body function. Its concern is the functional integrity of the musculoskeletal system. In addition to manual methods, chiropractors use physical therapy modalities exercise, health and nutritional guidance. Web: *chiroweb.com*

117

F. MATHIUS ALEXANDER TECHNIQUE These lessons help end improper use of neuromuscular system and bring body posture back into balance. Eliminates psycho-physical interferences, helps release long-held tension, and aids in re-establishing muscle tone. Web: *alexandertechnique.com*

FELDENKRAIS METHOD Dr. Moshe Feldenkrais founded this in the late 1940s. Lessons lead to improved posture and help create ease and efficiency of movement. This method is a great stress removal. Web: *feldenkrais.com*

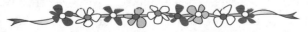

If you have mastered yourself, nature will obey you. – Eliphas Levi

Alternative Health Therapies & Massage Techniques

HOMEOPATHY In the 1800's, Dr. Samuel Hahnemann developed homeopathy. Patients are treated with minute amounts of substances similar to those that cause a particular disease to trigger the body's own defenses. The homeopathic principle is *Like Cures Like*. This safe and nontoxic remedy is the #1 alternative therapy in Europe and Britain because it is inexpensive, seldom has any side effects, and brings fast results. Web: *homeopathic.org*

NATUROPATHY Brought to America by Dr. Benedict Lust, M.D., this treatment uses diet, herbs, homeopathy, fasting, exercise, hydrotherapy, manipulation and sunlight. (Dr. Paul C. Bragg graduated from Dr. Lust's first School of Naturopathy in the U.S. Now 6 schools) Practitioners work with your body to restore health naturally. They reject surgery and drugs except as a last resort. Web: *naturopathic.org*

OSTEOPATHY The first School of Osteopathy was founded in 1892 by Dr. Andrew Taylor Still, M.D. There are now 15 U.S. colleges. Treatment involves soft tissue, spinal and body adjustments that free the nervous system from interferences that can cause illness. Healing by adjustment also includes good nutrition, physical therapies, proper breathing and good posture. Dr. Still's premise: if the body structure is altered or abnormal, then proper body function is altered and can cause pain and illness. Web: *osteopathic.org*

REFLEXOLOGY OR ZONE THERAPY Founded by Eunice Ingham, author of *Stories The Feet Can Tell*, inspired by a Bragg Health Crusade when she was 17. Reflexology helps the body and organs by removing crystalline deposits from reflex areas (nerve endings) of feet and hands through deep pressure massage. Primitive reflexology originated in China and Egypt and Native American Indians and Kenyans self-practiced it for centuries. Reflexology activates the body's flow of healing and energy by dislodging deposits. Visit Eunice Ingham and nephew Dwight Byer's web: *www.reflexology-usa.net*

SKIN BRUSHING daily is wonderful for circulation, toning, cleansing and healing. Use a dry vegetable brush (never nylon) and brush lightly. Helps purify lymph so it's able to detoxify your blood and tissues. Removes old skin cells, uric acid crystals and toxic wastes that come up through skin's pores. Use loofah sponge for variety in shower or tub.

Alternative Health Therapies & Massage Techniques

REIKI A Japanese form of massage that means "Universal Life Energy." Reiki helps the body to detoxify, then re-balance and heal itself. Discovered in the ancient Sutra manuscripts by Dr. Mikso Usui in 1822. Web: *reiki.org*

ROLFING Developed by Ida Rolf in the 1930's in the U.S. Rolfing is also called structural processing and postural release, or structural dynamics. It is based on the concept that distortions (accidents, injuries, falls, etc.) and the effects of gravity on the body cause upsets and long-term stress in the body. Rolfing helps to achieve balance and improved body posture. Methods involve the use of stretching, deep tissue massage, and relaxation techniques to loosen old injuries and break bad movement and posture patterns. Web: *rolf.org*

TRAGERING Founded by Dr. Milton Trager M.D., who was inspired at age 18 by Paul C. Bragg to become a doctor. It is a mind-body learning method that involves gentle shaking and rocking, allowing the body to let go, releasing tensions and lengthening the muscles for more body peace and health. Tragering can do miraculous healing where needed in the muscles and the entire body. Web: *trager.com*

119

WATER THERAPY Soothing detox shower: apply olive oil to skin, alternate hot and cold water, every 2-3 minutes. Massage body while under hot, filtered spray. Garden hose massage is great in summer or anytime. Hot detox soak bath (diabetics use warm water) 20 minutes with cup of Epsom salts or apple cider vinegar. This soak helps pull out the toxins by creating an artificial fever cleanse. Web: *holisticonline.com/hydrotherapy.htm*

MASSAGE & AROMATHERAPY works two ways: the essence (aroma) relaxes, as does the massage. Essential oils are extracted from flowers, leaves, roots, seeds and barks. These are usually massaged into the skin, inhaled or used in a bath for their ability to relax, soothe and heal. The oils, used for centuries to treat numerous ailments, are revitalizing and energizing for the body and mind. Example: Tiger balm, MSM, echinacea and arnica help relieve muscle aches. Avoid skin creams and lotions with mineral oil – it clogs the skin's pores. Use these natural oils for the skin: almond, apricot kernel, avocado, and I use Bragg Organic Olive Oil and mix with aromatic essential oils: rosemary, lavender, rose, jasmine, sandalwood, lemon-balm, etc. – 6 oz. oil and 6 drops of an essential oil. Web: *naha.org*

Alternative Health Therapies & Massage Techniques

MASSAGE – SELF Paul C. Bragg often said, "You can be your own best massage therapist, even if you have only one good hand." Near-miraculous health improvements have been achieved by victims of accidents or strokes in bringing life back to afflicted parts of their own bodies by self-massage and even vibrators. Treatments can be day or night, almost continual. Self-massage also helps achieve relaxation at day's end. Families and friends can learn and exchange massages; it's a wonderful sharing experience. Remember, babies love and thrive with daily massages, start from birth. Family pets also love soothing, healing touch of massages. Web: *coolnurse.com/massage.htm*

MASSAGE – SHIATSU Japanese form of health massage that applies pressure from the fingers, hands, elbows and even knees along the same points as acupuncture. Shiatsu has been used in Asia for centuries to relieve pain, common ills, muscle stress and to aid lymphatic circulation. Web: *shiatsu.org*

MASSAGE – SPORTS An important health support system for professional and amateur athletes. Sports massage improves circulation and mobility to injured tissue, enables athletes to recover more rapidly from myofascial injury, reduces muscle soreness and chronic strain patterns. Soft tissues are freed of trigger points and adhesions, thus contributing to improvement of peak neuro-muscular functioning and athletic performance.

MASSAGE – SWEDISH One of the oldest and the most popular and widely used massage techniques. This deep body massage soothes and promotes healthy circulation and is a great way to loosen and relax tight muscles before and after exercise. Web: *massageden.com/swedish-massage.shtml*

Author's Comment: We have personally sampled many of these Alternative Therapies. It's estimated that soon America's health care costs will leap over $2 trillion. It's more important than ever to be responsible for our own health! This includes seeking holistic health practitioners who are dedicated to keeping us well by inspiring us to practice prevention! These Alternative Healing Therapies are also popular and getting results: aroma, Ayurvedic, biofeedback, color, guided imagery, herbs, music, meditation, magnets, saunas, tai chi, chi gong, Pilates, Rebounder, yoga, etc. Explore them and be open to improving your earthly temple for a healthy, happier, longer life.

Seek and find the best for your body, mind and soul. – Patricia Bragg

A Personal Message to Our Students
The Body Self-Cleans & Self-Heals When Given A Chance

It is our sincere desire that each one of our readers and students attain this precious super health and enjoy freedom from all nagging, tormenting human ailments. After studying this healthy spine program, you know that most physical problems arise from an unhealthy lifestyle that creates toxins throughout the body. Many trouble spots are years old and are mainly concentrated in the intestines, colon and organs.

We have taught you that there is no special diet for any one special ailment! The Bragg Healthy Lifestyle promotes cleansing through the eating of more organic raw fruits and vegetables combined with regular fasting. It is only through progressive cleansing that the human "cesspool" can be banished! We have told you that you will go through healing crises from time to time. During these cleansing times you might have weakness and might become discouraged! This is the time you must have great strength and faith! It is during these crises, when you feel the worst, that you are doing the greatest amount of deep detox cleansing. This is why weaklings, crybabies and people without will-power and intestinal fortitude fail to follow this perfect Bragg Heathy Lifestyle System of Cleansing, Healing and Rejuvenation! Please be strong!

121

Weaklings want a cure that requires no effort on their part. Mother Nature and your body do not work that way! The average unfortunate sick person thinks of the Lord as a kind and forgiving Father who will allow them to enter the Garden of Eden effortlessly and unpunished for any violation of His and Mother Nature's Laws of Healthy Living.

You can create your own Garden of Eden anywhere you live, regardless of climate! All you have to do is to purify the body of its toxic poisons by living a healthy lifestyle. You can reach a stage of health and youthfulness that you never thought was possible! You can feel ageless where your chronological age actually stands still and pathological age will make you younger! When your body is free of deadly toxic material you will reach the physical, mental, emotional and spiritual state that will give you happiness every waking hour as it adds many more youthful, active, joyous years to your life!

You are not stuck where you are unless you decide to be. – Dr. Wayne Dyer

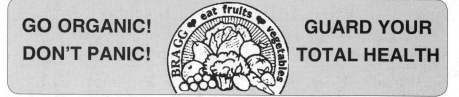

**GO ORGANIC!
DON'T PANIC!**

BRAGG • eat fruits • vegetables

**GUARD YOUR
TOTAL HEALTH**

FROM THE AUTHORS

This book was written for You! It can be your passport to a healthy, long, vital life. We in the Alternative Health Therapies join hands in one common objective – promoting a high standard of health for everyone. Healthy nutrition points the way – which is Mother Nature and God's Way. This book teaches you how to work with them, not against them! Health Doctors, Therapists Nurses, Teachers and Caregivers are becoming more dedicated than ever before to keeping their patients healthy and fit. This book was written to emphasize the great needed importance of living a lifetime of healthy living, close to Mother Nature and God.

Statements in this book are scientific health findings, known facts of physiology and biological therapeutics. Paul C. Bragg practiced natural methods of living for over 80 years with highly beneficial results, knowing that they were safe and of great value. His daughter Patricia lectured and co-authored the Bragg Health Books with him and continues to carrying on The Bragg Health Crusades.

Paul C. Bragg and daughter Patricia express their opinions solely as Public Health Educators and Health Crusaders. They offer no cure for disease. Only the body has the ability to cure a person. Experts may disagree with some of the statements made in this book. However, such statements are considered to be factual, based on the long-time experience of pioneer Health Crusaders Paul C. Bragg and Patricia Bragg. If you suspect you have a medical problem, please seek alternative health professionals to help you make the healthiest, wisest and best-informed choices!

Count your blessings daily while you do your 30 to 45 minute brisk walks and exercises with these affirmations – health! strength! youth! vitality! peace! laughter! humility! understanding! forgiveness! joy! and love for eternity!– and soon all these qualities will come flooding and bouncing into your life. With blessings of super health, peace and love to you, our dear friends – our readers. – Patricia Bragg

If I were to name the three most precious resources of life, I would say books, friends and nature; and the greatest of these, at least the most constant and always at hand is Mother Nature and God. – John Burroughs

Peace is not a season, it is a way of life, to enjoy each day.

Change your mind and you can change your life.

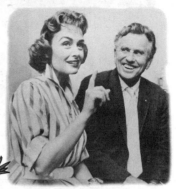

Thanks for The Bragg Healthy Lifestyle that you shared with me and are sharing with millions of others world-wide.
– John Gray, Ph.D., Author

Actress Donna Reed with Paul Bragg

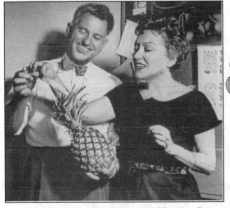

Paul Bragg, Creator of Health Food Stores, with his prize student Jack LaLanne, who thanks Bragg for saving his life at 15.

Thanks to Paul Bragg & Daughter Patricia for my easy to follow Health Program. You make my days healthy.– Clint Eastwood Bragg Follower for over 55 years.

PAUL BRAGG, N.D., Ph.D
Life Extension Specialist and Originator of Health Food Stores

In Medical School I read Dr. Bragg's Health Books and they changed my way of thinking and the path of my life. I founded the Omega Institute.
– Stephan Rechtschaffen, M.D.
www.eomega.org • famous since 1977

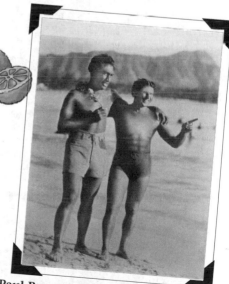

Paul Bragg with Actress Gloria Swanson who became a Bragg devotee when she was 18. She often health crusaded with Bragg.

I lost 102 lbs. with Bragg Apple Cider Vinegar and The Bragg Healthy Lifestyle and have kept it off for over 15 years, staying away from white flour, sugar and other processed foods. – Dee McCaffrey, Chemist & Diet Counselor, Tempe, AZ

Paul Bragg with Duke Kahanamoku, Olympic swimmer who taught Paul how to surf. His beautiful wife Nadine was Patricia's godmother.

123

The Bragg Healthy Lifestyle teaches you to be healthy, fit and ageless.
– Mark Victor Hansen, Co-Producer "Chicken Soup for the Soul" Series

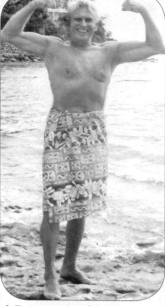

PAUL BRAGG STAYING HEALTHY AND FIT!

Paul C. Bragg in Tahiti gathering delicious tropical papaya fruits.

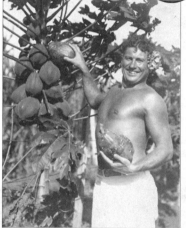

Paul Bragg owes his powerful body and superb health to living exclusively on live, vital, healthy, nutrient rich foods.

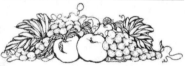

Paul C. Bragg and daughter Patricia were my early guiding inspiration to my education and health career.
– Jeffery Bland, Ph.D., Famous Food Scientist

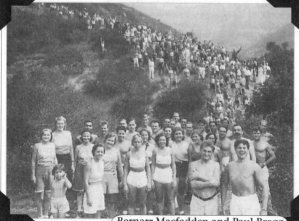

Bernarr Macfadden and Paul Bragg

A thousand happy Bragg Health Students enjoy hiking, exercise and fresh air on the trail to Mount Hollywood (above Griffith Observatory) in beautiful California, the summer of 1932.

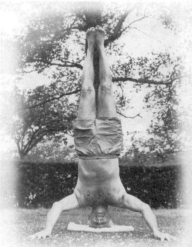

Paul Bragg at beautiful Regent's Park, London

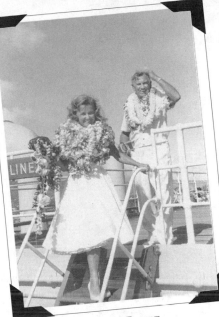

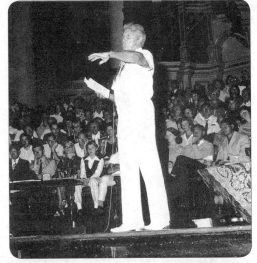

PAUL & PATRICIA BRAGG HEALTH CRUSADING SYDNEY, AUSTRALIA

Patricia and Paul Bragg on world trip in 1950's, during Tahiti stop.

During the 40-plus years Patricia worked with her father, she was right there beside him, assisting him on the Bragg Health Crusades world-wide. They were a team, when you looked at them, you would see only two people headed in the same direction.

Our lives have completely turned around! Our family is feeling so very healthy, we must tell you about it.– Gene & Joan Zollner, parents of 11, Bellingham, WA

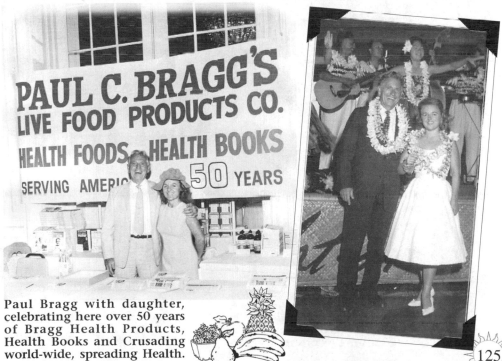

PAUL C. BRAGG'S
LIVE FOOD PRODUCTS CO.
HEALTH FOODS – HEALTH BOOKS
SERVING AMERIC[A] 50 YEARS

Paul Bragg with daughter, celebrating here over 50 years of Bragg Health Products, Health Books and Crusading world-wide, spreading Health.

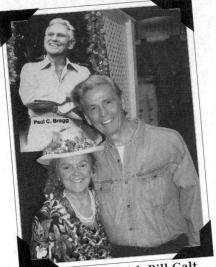

Patricia Bragg with Bill Galt
founder of Good Earth Restaurants

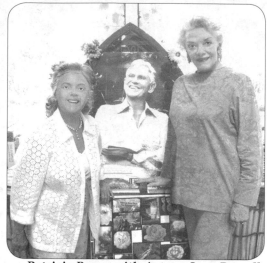

Patricia Bragg with Actress Jane Russell,
photo of Paul Bragg in background.

PATRICIA BRAGG
CONTINUING THE
HEALTH CRUSADE!

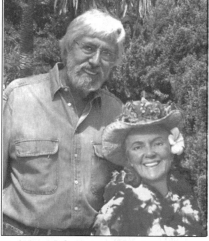

Patricia with Jean-Michel Cousteau
Ocean Explorer & Environmentalist

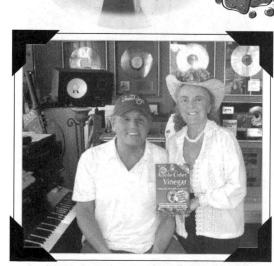

Patricia Bragg in the studio with
Beach Boy Bruce Johnson listening
to their latest song recordings.

Dear Friends – you can not know how greatly you have already impacted my life and some of my friends! We love your Bragg Health Books, teachings and products and are now living healthier, happier lives. Thanks! – Winnie Brown, Tucson, AZ

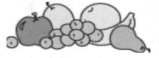

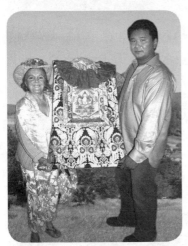

Patricia and Dali Lama's nephew,
Jigme Norbu presenting gift

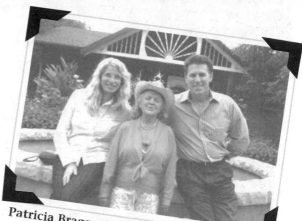

Patricia Bragg with Rev. Robert A. Schuller
and his wife Donna

No kind action ever
stops with itself.
One kind action
leads to another.
Good example is
followed. A single
act of kindness
throws out roots in
all directions, and
the roots spring up
and make new trees.
The greatest work that
kindness does to others is that
it makes them kind themselves.
– *Amelia Earhart, famous pilot*

Patricia with
Astronaut
Buzz Aldrin,
lunar pilot of
Apollo 11

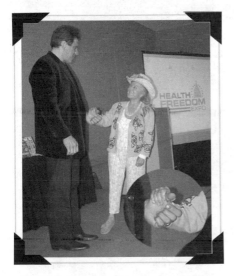

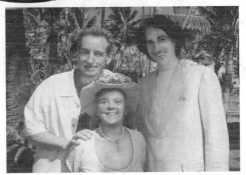

ABOVE: Patricia (center) with
Paul Wenner, Gardenburger Creator
(on left) and Dr. John Demartini,
star in *The Secret* (on right)
Both lives were blessed by Bragg Books

LEFT: Lou Ferrigno (the Incredible Hulk)
with Patricia Bragg speaking at the
Health Freedom Expo in Chicago.
Bragg Teachings inspired Lou.

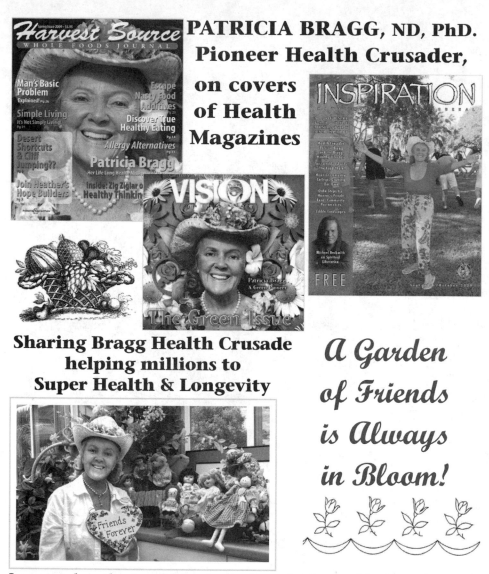

PATRICIA BRAGG, ND, PhD.
Pioneer Health Crusader,
on covers of Health Magazines

Sharing Bragg Health Crusade
helping millions to
Super Health & Longevity

A Garden
of Friends
is Always
in Bloom!

Love makes the world go 'round, and it's everlasting when it's given with caring, loving advice that will improve and enrich your life! This is why my father and I love sharing with you the health wisdoms which can be with you on your life's long healthy journey. We wish you all the peace, joy and happiness you need to have a long, fulfilling, healthy life.

With Love

Too often we underestimate the power of a kind touch, a warm smile, a kind word, a listening ear, an honest compliment, or the smallest act of caring, all of which have the potential to turn a life around. – Leo Buscaglia, Ph.D., Bragg Follower

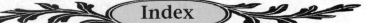

Perfect health is about gold; a sound body before riches. – Solomon

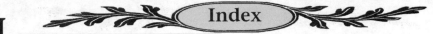

We are recharged and blessed by each one of you reading our health teachings and improving your health. Thank you. – Patricia Bragg

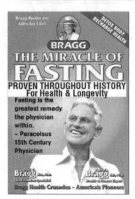
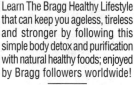
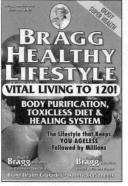
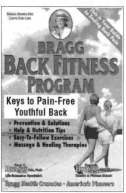
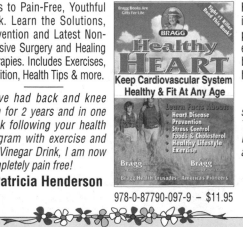

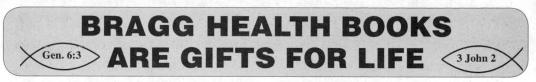
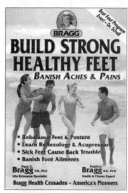
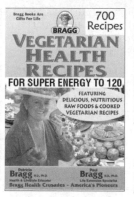
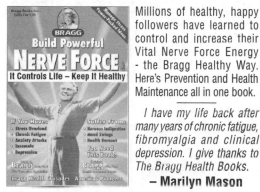
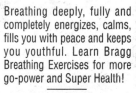

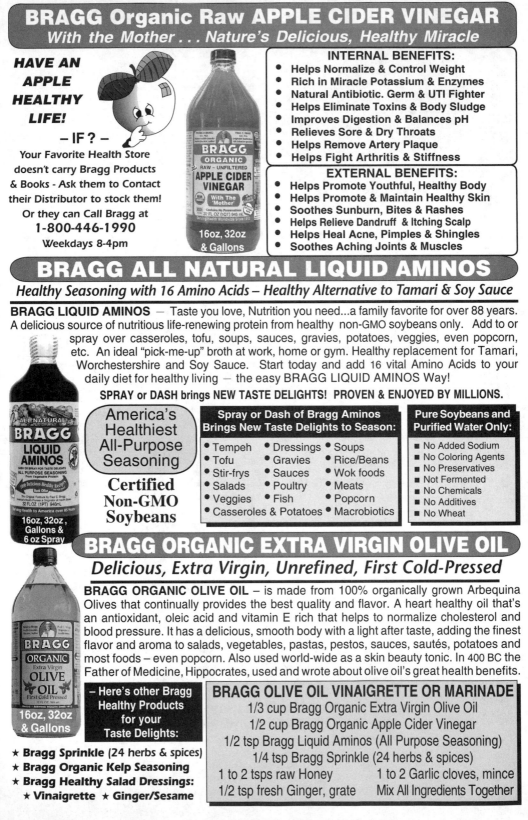

BRAGG ORGANIC APPLE CIDER VINEGAR

SIZE	PRICE	UPS SHIPPING & HANDLING For USA	$ Amount
16 oz.	$ 2.99 each	S/H – Please add $9. for 1st bottle and $1.50 each add'l bottle	
16 oz.	$ 33.00 Special Case /12	S/H Cost by Time Zone: CA $12. PST/MST $14. CST $22. EST $25	
32 oz.	$ 4.79 each	S/H – Please add $10. for 1st bottle – $2. each add'l bottle	
32 oz.	$ 52.00 Special Case /12	S/H Cost by Time Zone: CA $17. PST/MST $20. CST $35. EST $38	
1 gal.	$ 14.99 each	S/H – 1st bottle: CA $9. PST/MST $10. CST $13. EST $15 – $6. each add'l bottle	
1 gal.	$ 51.00 Special Case /4	S/H Cost by Time Zone: CA $17. PST/MST $20. CST $34. EST $37	

BRAGG Vinegar is a food and not taxable

BRAGG VINEGAR	$
(S&H) Shipping & Handling	
TOTAL	$

BRAGG LIQUID AMINOS

SIZE	PRICE	UPS SHIPPING & HANDLING For USA	$ Amount
6 oz.	$ 3.29 each	S/H – Please add $9. for 1st 3 bottles – $1.50 each add'l bottle	
6 oz.	$ 71.00 Special Case /24	S/H Cost by Time Zone: CA $10. PST/MST $11. CST $17. EST $19	
16 oz.	$ 4.29 each	S/H – Please add $9. for 1st bottle – $1.50 each add'l bottle	
16 oz.	$ 47.00 Special Case /12	S/H Cost by Time Zone: CA $12. PST/MST $14. CST $22. EST $25	
32 oz.	$ 6.99 each	S/H – Please add $10. for 1st bottle and $2. each add'l bottle	
32 oz.	$ 76.00 Special Case /12	S/H Cost by Time Zone: CA $17. PST/MST $20. CST $35. EST $38	
1 gal.	$ 25.79 each	S/H – 1st bottle: CA $9. PST/MST $10. CST $13. EST $15 – $6. each add'l bottle	
1 gal.	$ 88.00 Special Case /4	S/H Cost by Time Zone: CA $17. PST/MST $20. CST $34. EST $37	

BRAGG Aminos & Olive Oil are foods and not taxable

BRAGG AMINOS	$
(S&H) Shipping & Handling	
TOTAL	$

BRAGG ORGANIC OLIVE OIL

SIZE	PRICE	UPS SHIPPING & HANDLING For USA	$ Amount
16 oz.	$ 9.99 each	S/H – Please add $9. for 1st bottle – $1.50 each add'l bottle	
16 oz.	$ 108.00 Special Case /12	S/H Cost by Time Zone: CA $12. PST/MST $14. CST $22. EST $25	
32 oz.	$ 16.29 each	S/H – Please add $10. for 1st bottle and $2. each add'l bottle	
32 oz.	$ 176.00 Special Case /12	S/H Cost by Time Zone: CA $17. PST/MST $20. CST $35. EST $38	
1 gal.	$ 56.99 each	S/H – 1st bottle: CA $9. PST/MST $10. CST $13. EST $15 – $6. each add'l bottle	
1 gal.	$ 194.00 Special Case /4	S/H Cost by Time Zone: CA $17. PST/MST $20. CST $34. EST $37	

Please Specify: ☐ Check ☐ Money Order ☐ Cash
Charge to: ☐ Visa ☐ Master Card ☐ Discover
Credit Card Number:_____
Card Expires: _____ / _____ month / year

BRAGG OLIVE OIL	$
(S&H) Shipping & Handling	
TOTAL	$

VISA

MasterCard

DISCOVER

Signature:_____

Business office calls (805) 968-1020. We accept MasterCard, Discover & VISA phone orders. Please prepare order using order form. It speeds your call and serves as order record. Hours: 8 to 4 pm Pacific Time, Monday thru Thursday.
• Visit our Web: www.bragg.com • e-mail: bragg @ bragg.com

CREDIT CARD ORDERS
CALL (800) 446-1990
OR FAX (805) 968-1001

BOF 109

Mail to: **HEALTH SCIENCE, Box 7, Santa Barbara, CA 93102 USA**
Please Print or Type – Be sure to give street & house number to facilitate delivery.

Name _____
Address _____ Apt. No. _____
City _____ State _____ Zip _____
Phone ( ) _____ e-mail _____

Bragg Health Products available most Health Stores & Grocery Health Depts Nationwide

BRAGG HEALTHY SALAD DRESSINGS

✳ Organic Healthy Vinaigrette ✳ Made with Organic Ginger & Sesame

12 oz glass bottle

This Bragg Healthy Organic Vinaigrette Dressing makes a salad special with its tasty, tangy flavor. A zesty blend of our Bragg Organic Extra Virgin, First Cold Pressed Olive Oil, combined with our Bragg Organic Apple Cider Vinegar, Bragg Liquid Aminos, garlic, raw honey, onion, minced red bell peppers and delicious organic herbs. This unique taste brings you a healthy dressing with all the best of the Bragg tradition of healthy eating and living.

12 oz glass bottle

This Bragg Healthy Ginger Sesame Dressing is based on the delicious flavor of our famous Bragg Liquid Aminos. Ginger and Sesame Seeds are blended into our smooth, zesty dressing, then combined with Bragg Organic Extra Virgin Olive Oil, fresh garlic, raw honey, fresh ginger and lemon juice. Also delicious to spice up vegetable stir-frys, chicken or grilled vegetables. A sweet and tangy taste brings you the best of the Bragg tradition of healthy eating and living.

Made with ALL Bragg Healthy Ingredients

America's Healthiest All-Purpose Seasonings

BRAGG SPRINKLE ORGANIC 24 HERBS & SPICES

This old favorite is now available again. Bragg Sprinkle was created in 1931 by Paul C. Bragg, Health Pioneer and Originator of Health Food Stores. Organic Sprinkle adds new delicious healthy flavor to most recipes, meals and snacks. It's salt-free with no additives, preservatives or fillers.

Shaker Top

BRAGG ORGANIC SEA KELP DELIGHT
Feast of the Sea Seasoning

Shaker Top

This original Organic Kelp Seasoning made from sun-dried Organic Pacific Ocean Sea Kelp, combined with 24 all natural herbs & spices. It's a healthy, delicious seasoning for almost all recipes and meals and is specially suited for low sodium diets.

NEW BRAGG
Premium
NUTRITIONAL YEAST SEASONING

Provides great-taste and nutrition when added to a wide variety of foods. Sprinkle on salads, vegetables, potatoes, casseroles, soups, dips, spreads, and in juices and smoothies. Its "cheese-like" flavor makes it a 100% delicious, healthy seasoning. Nutritionally designed to help meet important nutritional needs of vegetarians, vegans and anyone wanting a good source of B12, B-Complex Vitamins.

Shaker Top

- Gluten-Free • Non-GMO
- No Salt • No Sugar • No Dairy
- No Artificial Colors & Preservatives
- No Brewery Products
- No Candida Albicans
- Vegetarian & Kosher Certified

You are what you eat, drink, breathe, think, say & do.
— Patricia Bragg, ND, PhD.

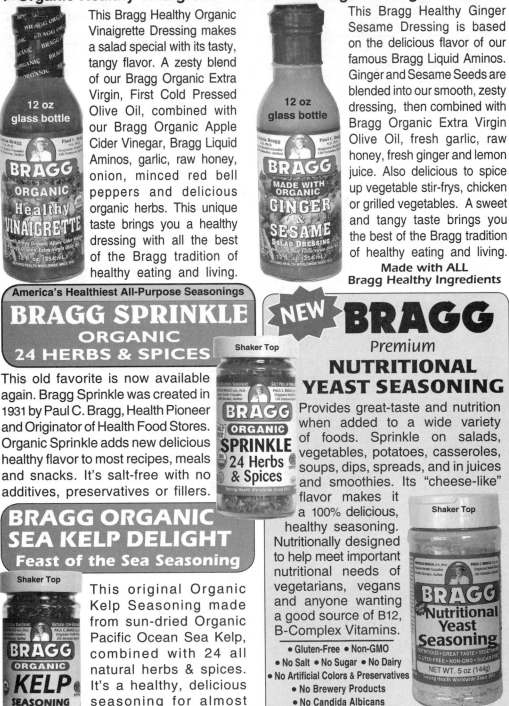

BRAGG SPRINKLE – 24 Herbs & Spices Seasoning

SIZE	PRICE		UPS SHIPPING & HANDLING For USA	$	Amount
1.5 oz.	$ 4.29	each	S/H – Please add $9. for 1st 3 bottles and $1. each add'l bottle		•
1.5 oz.	$ 47.00	Special Case /12	S/H Cost by Time Zone: CA $9. PST/MST $9. CST $10. EST $12.		•
BRAGG Sprinkle Seasoning is a food and not taxable			BRAGG SPRINKLE	$	•
			(S&H) Shipping & Handling		•
			TOTAL	$	•

BRAGG ORGANIC SEA KELP

SIZE	PRICE		UPS SHIPPING & HANDLING For USA	$	Amount
2.7 oz.	$ 4.29	each	S/H – Please add $9. for 1st 3 bottles and $1. each add'l bottle		•
2.7 oz.	$ 47.00	Special Case/12	S/H Cost by Time Zone: CA $9. PST/MST $9. CST $10. EST $12.		•
BRAGG Kelp Seasoning is a food and not taxable			BRAGG KELP	$	•
			(S&H) Shipping & Handling		•
			TOTAL	$	•

BRAGG NUTRITIONAL YEAST

SIZE	PRICE		UPS SHIPPING & HANDLING For USA	$	Amount
4.5 oz.	$ 5.69	each	S/H – Please add $9. for 1st 3 bottles and $1. each additional bottle		•
4.5 oz.	$ 63.00	Special Case /12	S/H Cost by Time Zone: CA $9. PST/MST $9. CST $10. EST $12.		•
BRAGG Nutritional Yeast Seasoning is a food and not taxable			BRAGG YEAST		
			(S&H) Shipping & Handling		•
			TOTAL	$	•

BRAGG SALAD DRESSINGS

SIZE	PRICE		UPS SHIPPING & HANDLING For USA	$	Amount
✱ BRAGG GINGER & SESAME SALAD DRESSING					
12 oz.	$ 4.99	each	S/H – Please add $9. for 1st bottle and $1.25 each add'l bottle		•
12 oz.	$ 54.00	Special Case /12	S/H Cost by Time Zone: CA $11. PST/MST $12. CST $19. EST $22.		•
✱ BRAGG ORGANIC VINAIGRETTE SALAD DRESSING					
12 oz.	$ 4.99	each	S/H – Please add $9. for 1st bottle and $1.25 each add'l bottle		•
12 oz.	$ 54.00	Special Case /12	S/H Cost by Time Zone: CA $11. PST/MST $12. CST $19. EST $22.		•
BRAGG Salad Dressings are foods and not taxable			BRAGG SALAD DRESSINGS	$	•
			(S&H) Shipping & Handling		•
			TOTAL	$	•

Payment Method:

☐ Check   ☐ Money Order   ☐ Cash

Charge To: ☐ Visa   ☐ Master Card   ☐ Discover

Credit Card Number:_____

Card Expires:_____ / _____
month / year

Signature:_____

Business office calls (805) 968-1020. We accept MasterCard, Discover & VISA phone orders. Please prepare order using order form. It speeds your call and serves as order record. Hours: 8 to 4 pm Pacific Time, Monday thru Thursday.
• Visit our Web: www.bragg.com • e-mail: bragg @ bragg.com

CREDIT CARD ORDERS
CALL (800) 446-1990
OR FAX (805) 968-1001

BOF 109

Mail to: **HEALTH SCIENCE, Box 7, Santa Barbara, CA 93102 USA**
Please Print or Type – Be sure to give street & house number to facilitate delivery.

Name _____

Address _____   Apt. No. _____

City _____   State _____   Zip _____

Phone ( ) _____   e-mail _____

Bragg Products available most Health Stores & Grocery Health Depts Nationwide

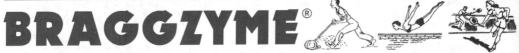
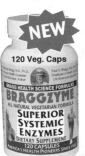

BRAGG ORGANIC APPLE CIDER VINEGAR DRINK

Apple Cider Vinegar & Honey

More organic, delicious Apple Cider Vinegar Drinks to come.
Please call our office for more information on flavors available.

SIZE	PRICE	QUANTITY	SHIP TO: CA	PST/MST	CST	EST	$ Amount
16 oz.	$ 2.19 each	1-2 bottles	$8.00	$8.00	$9.00	$12.00	•
16 oz.		3-4 bottles	$8.00	$9.00	$11.00	$13.00	•
16 oz.		5-6 bottles	$9.00	$9.00	$13.00	$15.00	•
16 oz.		7-12 bottles	$11.00	$13.00	$21.00	$24.00	•
16 oz.	$ 24.00	Special Case /12	$11.00	$13.00	$21.00	$24.00	•

**BRAGG APPLE CIDER VINEGAR DRINK
is a Food and is not taxable**

BRAGG VINEGAR DRINK $	•
(S&H) Shipping & Handling	•
TOTAL $	•

BRAGGZYME – Systemic Enzymes

SIZE	PRICE		UPS SHIPPING & HANDLING For USA	$ Amount
120 cap	$ 39.95	each	S/H – Please add $9. for 1st 3 bottles and $1. each add'l bottle	•
120 cap	$ 439.00	Special Case /12	S/H Cost by Time Zone: CA $9. PST/MST $9. CST $10. EST $12.	•

on Braggzyme CA only pays tax

for BRAGGZYME only CA Residents add 8.75% TAX $	•
(S&H) Shipping & Handling	•
TOTAL $	•

Payment Method:

☐ Check ☐ Money Order ☐ Cash

Charge To: ☐ Visa ☐ Master Card ☐ Discover

Credit Card
Number:_____

Card
Expires:_____ / _____
month / year

Signature:_____

VISA

MasterCard

DISCOVER

Business office calls (805) 968-1020.
We accept MasterCard, Discover & VISA.
Phone orders please prepare order using order forms,
as it speeds up your call and serves as order record.
Hours: 8 to 4 pm Pacific Time, Monday thru Thursday.
• Visit our Web: www.bragg.com • e-mail: bragg @ bragg.com

CREDIT CARD ORDERS
CALL (800) 446-1990
OR FAX (805) 968-1001

BOF 109

Mail to: **HEALTH SCIENCE, Box 7, Santa Barbara, CA 93102 USA**
Please Print or Type – Be sure to give street & house number to facilitate delivery.

Name

Address   **Apt. No.**

City   **State**   **Zip**

( )

Phone   **e-mail**

Bragg Products available most Health Stores & Grocery Health Depts Nationwide

— Make copies when needed for mailing in. —

Send for Free Health Bulletins

Patricia Bragg wants to keep in touch with you, your relatives and friends about the latest Health, Nutrition, Exercise and Longevity Discoveries. Please enclose one stamp for each USA name listed. Foreign listings send postal reply coupons.

With Blessings of Health, Peace and Thanks *Patricia*

Please make copy, then print clearly and mail to:

BRAGG HEALTH CRUSADES, Box 7, Santa Barbara, CA 93102

Name

Address   Apt. No.

City   State   Zip

Phone ( )   e-mail

Name

Address   Apt. No.

City   State   Zip

Phone ( )   e-mail

Name

Address   Apt. No.

City   State   Zip

Phone ( )   e-mail

Name

Address   Apt. No.

City   State   Zip

Phone ( )   e-mail

Name

Address   Apt. No.

City   State   Zip

Phone ( )   e-mail

Bragg Health Crusades spreading health worldwide since 1912

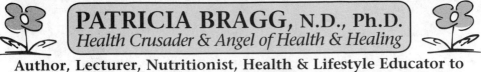

PATRICIA BRAGG, N.D., Ph.D.
Health Crusader & Angel of Health & Healing

Author, Lecturer, Nutritionist, Health & Lifestyle Educator to World Leaders, Hollywood Stars, Singers, Dancers, Athletes, etc.

Patricia is a 100% dedicated health crusader with a passion like her father, Paul C. Bragg, world renowned health authority. Patricia has won international fame on her own in this field. She conducts Bragg Health and Fitness Seminars for Conventions and Women's, Men's, Youth and Church Groups around the world and promotes Bragg Healthy Lifestyle Living and "How-To, Self-Health" Books on Radio and TV Talk Shows throughout the English-speaking world. Consultants to Presidents and Royalty, to Stars of Stage, Screen and TV and to Champion Athletes, Patricia and her father co-authored The Bragg Health Library of Instructive, Inspiring Books that promote a healthier lifestyle, for a long, healthy, happy life.

Patricia herself is the symbol of health, perpetual youthfulness and feminine, radiant, super energy. She is a living and sparkling example of her and her father's healthy lifestyle precepts and this she loves sharing world-wide.

A fifth-generation Californian on her mother's side, Patricia was reared by The Bragg Natural Health Method from infancy. In school, she not only excelled in athletics, but also won honors for her studies and her counseling. She is an accomplished musician and dancer . . . as well as tennis player and mountain climber . . . and the youngest woman ever to be granted a U.S. Patent. Patricia is a popular gifted Health Teacher and a dynamic, in-demand Talk Show Guest on Radio and TV where she regularly spreads the simple, easy-to-follow Bragg Healthy Lifestyle for everyone of all ages.

Man's body is his vehicle through life, his earthly temple . . . and the Creator wants us filled with joy & health for a long fruitful life. The Bragg Crusades of Health and Fitness (3 John 2) has carried her around the world over 15 times – spreading physical, emotional, mental and spiritual health and joy. Health is our birthright and Patricia teaches how to prevent the destruction of our health from man-made wrong lifestyle habits of living.

Patricia's been a Health Consultant to American Presidents, British Royalty, to Champion Triathletes and Betty Cuthbert, Australia's "Golden Girl," (16 world records and 4 Olympic track gold medals) and New Zealand's Olympic Track and Triathlete Star, Allison Roe. Among those who come to her for advice are some of Hollywood's top Stars from Clint Eastwood to the ever-youthful singing group, The Beach Boys and their families, Singing Stars of the Metropolitan Opera and top Ballet Stars. Patricia's message is of world-wide appeal to people of all ages, nationalities and walks-of-life. Those who follow The Bragg Healthy Lifestyle and attend the Bragg Crusades world-wide are living testimonials . . . like ageless, super athlete, Jack LaLanne, who at age 15 went from sickness to Total Health!